On Becoming a Mother

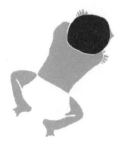

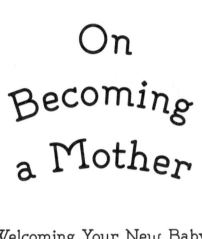

On Becoming a Mother

Welcoming Your New Baby
& Your New Life
with Wisdom from
around the World

Brigid McConville

ONEWORLD

A Oneworld Book

First published in Great Britain, North America, Australia and
the Commonwealth by Oneworld Publications 2014

ISBN 978-1-78074-389-9

Cover design by Anna Morrison
Printed and bound in Great Britain by
TJ International Ltd, Padstow, Cornwall

Acknowledgements and contributor credits appear on p. 273-7;
art credits appear on p. 278-81, which serve as a continuation of this page.

All recipes appearing in this book have been submitted by contributors and the
author and publisher make no claim to their accuracy or safety.

Proceeds from royalties on this book will support White Ribbon Alliance
(www.whiteribbonalliance.org).

Oneworld Publications
10 Bloomsbury Street, London WC1B 3SR, England

*To my mother Beryl, whose long life reached a peaceful end
during the writing of this book.*

*To Spike, an amazingly beautiful bundle of energy,
whose new life began.*

*To John, who got me into this motherhood lark
in the first place, and to our children Maeve, Arthur and Rory,
who would prefer not to be reminded of that.*

CONTENTS

PART 3: AFTER BIRTH

PART 4: THE "FIRST" YEAR

INTRODUCTION

Welcome to a world that you know or suspect is out there; a world in which women are celebrated, honoured, respected, admired and cared for as we become mothers.

At first glance, different parts of this world look dramatically different. In one country, birth happens between the white walls of a hospital; in another, women gather around the birthing woman singing in the dark of a hut, far from medical help.

But the woman at the centre of the picture – wherever she lives – is undertaking the same awesome journey to the edge of existence and back.

In one country, the image of her safe return, babe in arms, caught between tears and smiles, is shared via text message to all the friends on her partner's phone. In another, the good news is spread house to house by delighted dancing relatives, or solemnly announced to the Four Winds by an elder of the family. But everywhere there is relief and joy. She has returned – bringing new life – and she has changed. She has become a mother.

For the next few weeks, or even months in some enlightened places, the new mother and her baby are special. They need and deserve rest, nourishment, love and affection. Friends and relatives want to visit. They bring traditional food, gifts and good wishes. They embrace mother and child, offering wisdom and support as the child embarks on his or her first feed, first bath, first steps...

Of course, it is not always like that. And this book began from quite another starting place: the life-threatening neglect of pregnant women and mothers around the world, which the White Ribbon Alliance network advocates so passionately to change.

This book has been a wonderfully rewarding quest to the flip side of that neglect. It is full of inspiring stories that show how pregnancy and birth should be – and is, for many. We draw our energy to change things for all mothers from that knowledge of how it ought to be, and one day will be.

Brigid McConville

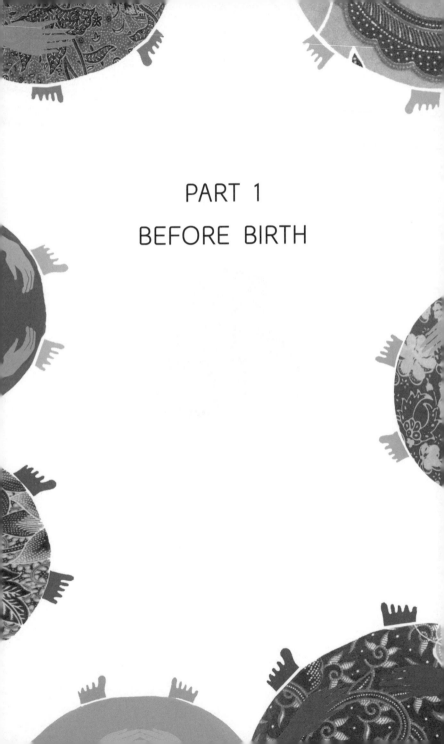

PART 1
BEFORE BIRTH

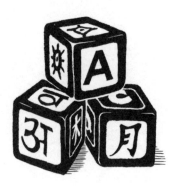

1

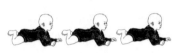

SHARING THE NEWS:
SHAAD (BANGLADESH)

When is the "right" time to tell the world that you are expecting a baby?

The answer differs from place to place, but there is a common theme to the timing of the announcement. Whether you live in the UK or the USA, where women tend to wait three months (since the risk of miscarriage diminishes after the first trimester), or in Bangladesh, where women wait seven months (by which time the baby has a much better chance of surviving an early birth), people express worry about "tempting fate" or attracting the "evil eye" by sharing the news or preparing for the baby too soon.

Even where women and babies are most likely to do well, families and friends commonly delay buying gifts until the baby has safely arrived.

But what all cultures have in common is a tremendous surge of celebration once the pregnancy is official.

The first signs

Dr Shabnam Shahnaz grew up in Dhaka, Bangladesh, one of five children in her family – four girls and one boy. She met her husband while they were both students in medical college. "Mine was the first 'love marriage' in my immediate family," she says. "My paternal grandmother was very upset about this, but my father and mother defended my choice and said they wanted me to be happy."

Soon after their marriage, Shabnam got pregnant. "It felt like a great miracle as I had been told that due to a previous health problem I could never have a baby. My husband and I were absolutely thrilled. This baby was so wanted!

"We kept quiet about it until the fourth month, when I finally told my close family and my mother-in-law. We were living in the house with my in-laws and I needed my mother-in-law to know why I was sleeping so much and why I was so hungry. Usually a daughter-in-law is expected to be up and helping at the breakfast table, but once she knew I was pregnant I was excused duties and encouraged to sleep in. This was her first grandchild, and from this early stage I felt well looked after."

A time to be doted on

"In Bangladesh, we formally announce we are having a baby only when we have reached the seventh month. Our belief is that by this time the baby is strong and will survive any sort of 'evil eye'; it's also scientifically true that by this time a baby is viable and can often survive on its own if the mother gives birth early.

"In accordance with tradition, my mother then told her brother, who is my uncle. They next arranged a date for the pregnancy ceremony, and invited my aunts, cousins and siblings, and all of my husband's family too," Shabnam says.

"A lot of food was cooked in my mother's house, and each of the guests brought a special dish that they knew I would really like. I was given many gifts, including jewellery and a new sari from my husband."

It was almost like a wedding.
– Shabnam Shahnaz, Bangladesh

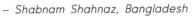

"It was such a nice feeling to be together celebrating with all of the people I knew I could rely on in the future. If anything should go wrong they would be the ones to help me; if all went well they would be celebrating with us."

Life-saving support

"I knew I was responsible for this new life, but I was just taking care of things blindly, not knowing what might go wrong, even with my medical training," remembers Shabnam, a member of White Ribbon Alliance Bangladesh who now lives and works in London.

"I felt vulnerable and scared. And indeed when I had a C-section and urgently needed blood, the group of people who had attended my party were the ones who immediately offered help," she says. "I have a rare blood group but within an hour they had found two blood donors for me. I come from an urban area, but the same traditions are strong in the rural areas of Bangladesh – and imagine what a lifesaver they must be for so many women.

"Sadly I miscarried my second child at five months and that was very hard, because I had not reached the seventh month and so I could not share my loss with many others. And so, with my third pregnancy, it was a big relief when I got to the seventh month – and it was time for another ceremony. I was working full-time as a doctor by then, tired and not eating well, but the pregnancy ceremony reminded me that I had a big responsibility and it was important for me to take care of myself.

"On the days of those pregnancy ceremonies I felt so cherished and protected, with people taking time to share their experiences and talk with me. It was so important for me and for my child to feel assured of a place in the community even before he or she was born. There was a lot of love; it was one of the happiest days of my life. This is something that every pregnant woman should have."

✳ ✳ ✳ ✳

The first welcoming

It can be hard for women and their partners to find time to fully acknowledge and accept the changes that a new pregnancy will bring to their life.

In Sufi tradition, a person undertakes a *muraqaba* (مراقبة, or watching), as a way of caring for the soul – or "looking over" it, which is the direct translation of the Arabic. This Sufi-inspired meditation is intended to provide a space in which to welcome your new child, before you announce your pregnancy to your larger family and community of friends:

- ✧ Sit face to face with your partner in a quiet place and hold hands.
- ✧ Close your eyes and draw your attention and your awareness to your heart (*qalb*) and how you are feeling about the baby. Think of your heart as a container for these feelings.
- ✧ In your mind's eye, connect the feelings of your heart with that of your partner, and with the energy of the growing baby, which lies between you.
- ✧ Summon thoughts of love and welcome, shared among the baby, your partner and yourself, and remember and call forth these feelings when you need sustenance during the months of change ahead.

What expecting really means

From *exspectare*, Latin for 'to look out for'

"Big belly" is the term for a pregnant woman, and pregnancy is the "big belly business", in the slang of Liberia. The term is used with affection and respect; women who are pregnant are openly referred to as "big belly" by midwives and doctors. A maternal waiting home may have the phrase "House for Big Belly to Stay Before Delivery" painted along one side, and public health posters exhort that "Every big belly must be tested for HIV".

A "big belly" is one visible sign to the world of a coming baby, so it's not surprising to find it used to identify women who are expecting. The Spanish use the phrase *estar preñada* ("to be big with young"), while *bombo* ("swollen") is often heard in Mexico. Cantonese slang labels you as a *da du po* (大肚, "big stomach woman"). And linguist Mark Peters, who writes for *McSweeney's* and *Visual Thesaurus*, says the term "clergy of belly" means something akin to "Come on, I'm pregnant, cut me some slack here" – a way of asking for mercy from the laws of the Church during pregnancy. It appeared in English by the seventeenth century.

Baking and cooking something up is a common theme around the globe. The phrase "in the pudding club" is recorded in *Barrere & Leland's Dictionary of Slang* (1890), while the related baking metaphor "up the duff" (*duff* being a boiled or steamed flour pudding) first shows up in *John Baker's Dictionary of Australian Slang* in 1941. In France, you have *une brioche au four* ("a brioche in the oven"), while the Germans have *einen Braten in den Ofen* ("a roast in the oven").

Since 1812, "Mr Knap is concerned" has been an oblique way to indicate pregnancy, according to *Green's Dictionary of Slang*. "Mr Knap" alludes to a woman having been knapped or knocked up. In France, rather than knocking things together, you are *en cloque* ("blistered"). These evocative terms may soon be overtaken by "SMEP", internet slang for a "sperm-meets-egg plan". Pregnancy is about worlds colliding, in any case.

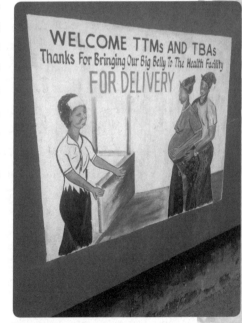

Welcoming trained traditional midwives and traditional birth attendants to a "Big Belly House" in Liberia

2

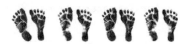

FINDING SUPPORT:
THE *HARAOBI* (JAPAN)

In a practice dating back to the eighth century, Japanese women wear a *haraobi*, or belly (*hara* 腹) sash (*obi* 帯), when they are pregnant. Wakako Kai, new mother of a baby girl, Mei, recalls: "My husband and mother-in-law took me to a shrine and prayed for my safe delivery; they bought the *haraobi* at the shrine. The *haraobi* is traditionally bought at a shrine since it is believed to have spiritual significance. It is the job of the mother of the pregnant daughter to buy it, but in my case my mother is living far from where I live. I was also given a charm for safe delivery, called an *omamori*, when I was given the sash."

Unlike other sashes in Japan, the *haraobi* is worn under the kimono, next to the skin. A strip of cotton or silk about twelve feet long and seven inches wide, it is typically red or white – auspicious colours. Traditionally, the sash was adorned with images of dogs, because it was believed that dogs gave birth easily. Women usually begin wearing the *haraobi* on the "day of the dog" at the beginning of their fifth month, when they have felt the first "quickening" or stirrings of the baby. For this reason, it has been a marker that the time of greatest risk of losing the baby has passed.

The *haraobi* is wrapped three times around the woman by her relatives or her midwife, making this a ritual shared by those supporting the mother. A monk (or, these days, the doctor) inscribes it with the *kanji* character for happiness (幸福). It has long been seen as a way of calling upon spiritual powers to hold the baby in place, with its head down, to prevent it from moving about too much. It is said that the *haraobi* helps to hold the spirit of the child in place too.

"I got my *haraobi* on the day of the dog during my fifth month of pregnancy," Wakako says. "Mine was a white cotton *haraobi*; most of them these days are made of cotton since it is washable and absorbent. Mothers can also reuse them to make things for the baby after the birth."

The material may be used to wrap other presents for the mother, to suggest that the pregnancy itself is precious and must be cared for.

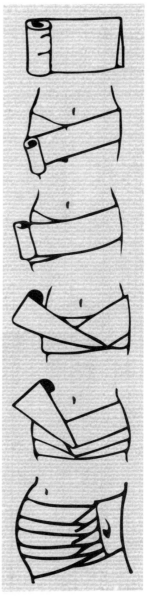

Tying a *haraobi*

Like pregnancy sashes worn in other countries, the *haraobi* also serves a practical end: to give back support, comfort and warmth.

"Although this is an ancient tradition, maternity clothing and underwear manufacturers have invented many good pregnancy sashes that suit the modern lifestyle," Wakako explains. "Many pregnant women, like me, put their ceremonial *haraobi* from the shrine in a drawer and wear a modern one instead!

"As with many other religions around the world, most Japanese people do not follow the rituals of the Shinto shrines any more – except when they feel that their health or their lives are at risk! And, like the majority of Japanese women, I feel that these days the *haraobi* ritual is more cultural than spiritual. However, I also feel it was good that my mother-in-law bought me the *haraobi* and the *omamori*. Maybe thanks to that mine was a very safe delivery and my baby girl is growing up healthy."

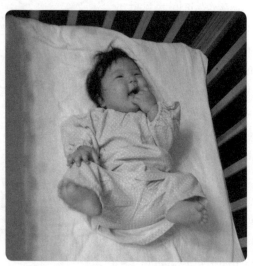

Wakako's daughter Mei

A sign of respect

Two weeks after the baby's birth, the mother and her husband will take the newborn to meet the husband's father or grandfather. In our culture, it is the grandfather or father-in-law or the husband's sister (auntie) who gives the child his or her clan name.

The husband's family will prepare by slaughtering a sheep or goat or, if they are rich, a cow. There will be much celebrating and eating, and the child will be given the name dedicated to his or her ancestors with a blessing.

At this time, the grandfather will thank the new mother for carrying the child during the long months of pregnancy. The father-in-law will give the baby a gift – a cow or goat or chicken. These days, friends and relatives will also give the baby clothes or cash.

Most important, the husband must buy his wife a new sash, called a *gomesi* or *busuuti*. This is traditional attire, an important piece of clothing worn at special functions such as weddings and funerals. This sash is a sign of appreciation for what his wife has been through.

It is an exciting moment and makes the woman feel cared for and loved by all.

– Samuel Senfuka, a chief of the Buganda people, Uganda

3

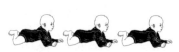

FOR SAFE KEEPING:
"SECRET MOTHERS" (MALAWI)

Chief Mac Julio Kwataine Masina is one of Malawi's twenty thousand chiefs. As a senior chief, he oversees eighty-nine villages in a sizeable area called Kwataine in Ntcheu District, which is home to half a million people – many of whom are Ngoni, and proudly trace their lineage to the once dominant Zulu nation.

Many years ago, he had watched as a woman in labour struggled to give birth. A traditional birth attendant was helping her, and in her opinion the woman had been subjected to witchcraft – an old belief among the Ngoni. No one in his village knew what to do. Finally, after more than twelve hours in labour, some men decided to carry her to the nearest hospital, despite the resistance of the village's leader. Still, she died before they got there. "I saw it with my own eyes," he says. After he became chief in 2000, he told the people of Kwataine that he "would never let a woman die during a traditional birth".

Care by committee

Indeed, the Chief has made the care of pregnant women everyone's business in Kwataine, by setting up some fifty "safe motherhood committees".

A hallmark of the Chief's committees are the *azimayi a chinsisi*, or "secret mothers", older women who introduce the expecting mother to local health workers, and help to cement the relationship, starting from the moment the pregnancy becomes known and lasting until forty days after the baby's birth.

This has proved a groundbreaking initiative, because, in Ngoni culture, it is not done to share news of your pregnancy with anyone other than your own mother. Men generally decide when a member of their family should go to a health centre or hospital, and there is a strong belief that children should be born at home. These traditions have meant that many young women have often gone without professional health care, giving birth with only the help of an unskilled attendant, just like their own mother and grandmothers.

Now, under the Chief's direction, when a woman becomes pregnant she must report her pregnancy to a local secret mother who takes charge of her health. It is the secret mother's duty to ensure that the woman goes to antenatal care appointments, gives birth with professional care in a health centre and receives vital postnatal care.

Immediately, the secret mothers were a success. Since 2006, no women have been reported to have died while giving birth in Kwataine villages. In 2012, Malawi's president, Joyce Banda, launched the Presidential Initiative in Safe Motherhood and named Masina as its chair. Lennie Kamwendo, a commissioner for health in Malawi and a leader of White Ribbon Alliance, says, "Women in Ntcheu District now use health facilities for childbirth more than ever before because of the Chief's efforts on safe motherhood, coupled with the government's ban on traditional birth attendants assisting in deliveries."

> A woman has a right to life and also a right to health. Why should women die like goats? Because they want to give life?
> *– Chief Kwataine, Ntcheu District, Malawi*

Help to carry the heavy loads

Masina insists that men in Kwataine be active in his safe motherhood programmes too. Village leaders must ensure that women's rights are protected, especially while they are pregnant. Those who do not do this can be fined – in some cases, forced to pay a goat or a chicken, the equivalent of a huge sum for a working farmer. Those who show support for the initiative are rewarded with chivalry, receiving a bead from Chief Kwataine's regalia. He explains: "To get a bead worn by the Chief in our culture means a life uplifted."

To the north of Malawi, in Uganda, men are also in the spotlight when it comes to supporting women during pregnancy. Fred Musoke is the director of the Community Health Empowerment Organization of Luwero, about eighty kilometres from the nation's capital, Kampala. Himself a father of four, he believes "a baby in the family concretes the relationship of the married couple, and the family at large. Having a baby here in Africa is seen as

The woman is pampered

In Igboland, when a woman gets pregnant, everyone around her gets so happy. As soon as the signs of pregnancy are seen, everything changes for the woman, from her eating habits to her style of dress.

We consider pregnancy as very delicate, so the woman is pampered. She must stop doing stressful domestic chores, and family members, friends and neighbours always come around to help and make sure that nothing harms the pregnancy. Old women sing songs and entertain the pregnant woman to be sure she is relaxed in mind and body. This helps avoid raised blood pressure, because we know this is bad for the pregnancy.

The traditional red *uhie*, yellow *odo* and black *uri* powders may be given to the woman by her birth attendant. Some are used for their decorative purposes, others to aid in healing.

Family members also prepare special delicacies to nourish the woman and the developing baby in the womb. As the saying goes in Igboland, *Ihe na agu Nwayi di ime na agu onye tuwara ya ime* – "Whatever a pregnant woman desires, the man who got her pregnant wants too."

– *Lizzy Agams, Igbo people, Nigeria*

a great privilege." He goes on: "People will come with gifts like clothes, chickens, goats, even cows, to show their encouragement and appreciation. The mother should always be given great wealth, because we expect much from her and she plays a big role in expanding the family."

However, Fred is highly critical of those of his fellow countrymen who neglect their responsibilities as fathers. During pregnancy, "the responsible father should help his wife to carry any heavy loads. He should fetch the water, cut the firewood, escort her to the nearest health facilities and encourage her to take any medications as directed by her health worker. The good father should also show care and love to the mother of his coming child. He should avoid harassing her and be sharing."

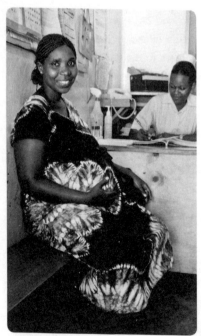

Expecting mother at clinic, Uganda

A new job

Of course, the father's role is just beginning in these days. He will have more to do once the contractions come. Fred continues: "During the time of birth, he should attend his wife, pay any hospital bills and buy nourishing food for her. And, after the baby is born, he should help the mother with the care of the baby, buying clothes for mother and child, saving for school fees, paying for any health treatments and making sure that immunizations are completed."

> As a father he must teach and guide his children, the "good morrow" must be practised and child rights respected.
>
> — *Fred Musoke, Uganda*

Says Fred, "Some families in Luwero have been abandoned by their fathers, the reason being that so many children are too much of a drain on his income – like one woman, Rose Nabukenya, raising seven children under ten years of age. They are the vulnerable people in my community."

Luwero's Community Health Empowerment Organization educates men in the community to understand their roles and responsibilities, from making the decision with his wife to expand the family, to finding ways to earn extra income to support extra children.

Kupadi: Dishing up support

"When I came to southern India mid-way through my pregnancy, I experienced the support and affection of my women friends and family through the Kodava people's custom of *kupadi*," says Dr Radha Karnad, who now lives in Nairobi. In her novel *The Scent of Pepper*, surgeon Kavery Nambisan notes that *kupadi* was meant to ensure a pregnant woman remained healthy during and after childbirth. "Eggs laid by red hens, ladles of ghee, and akki otti with wild honey" – a savoury rice pancake – were often served.

Radha remembers that "many brought my favourite foods for me – to my delight, these were all supposed to be dishes containing meat". She has a special fondness for Kodavathi *pandi kari*.

Pandi Kari (Spiced Pork)

Ingredients

2¼ lbs (1 kg) pork with skin and fat, cut into small pieces
salt
1 tsp fresh ground black pepper
1 tsp turmeric
6 medium onions, sliced
1 whole head of garlic, peeled and coarsely crushed
2 inch piece of ginger, crushed
3 level tbsp coriander powder
2 level tbsp chilli powder
kachampuli (extract of garcinia fruit), to taste
(malt vinegar can be substituted)
1 tsp *jeera* (cumin) seeds
½ tsp mustard seeds
cooking oil

Method

Wash the pork and drain (keeping aside ½ cup of the water); rub the meat with 1 tsp each of salt, pepper and turmeric. Combine the sliced onions and crushed garlic with the pork. Heat about 3 tbsp of oil over a medium heat in a saucepan; add the crushed ginger and fry until brown. Add the browned ginger to the pork. Reduce to low heat, add the coriander while stirring continuously for about 1 minute. Then add the chilli powder and stir until the mixture turns coffee brown. Add the pork and ½ cup of water. Cover and cook over medium heat until all the water evaporates, stirring occasionally. Add warm water to just cover the meat, and cook uncovered until the pork is done. Then add about 1 tsp of *kachampuli*, stir and cook for a further 5 to 10 minutes on low heat. Taste and add salt or *kachampuli* to taste. The oil should be rising to the surface. Roast the cumin and mustard seeds on a hot *tava* (griddle) or pan until medium brown; cool and then grind to a fine powder. Add the ground *jeera* and mustard seeds to the curry. Serves 6 to 8. ✖ ✖ ✖ ✖

✖ ✖ ✖ ✖ ✖ ✖ ✖ ✖ ✖ ✖ ✖ ✖

Rodent revenge

In Moldova it is thought that when a pregnant woman asks you for something, you should grant her wish — or risk having mice eat your clothes!

— *Ionela Bodrug*

4

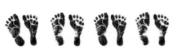

THE *HÓZHÓJÍ*:
MAKING A BLESSINGWAY (NAVAJO)

At the centre of the Navajo creation myth is *Asdzán Nádlééhé*, Changing Woman, who is seen in many ways to be the "inner form" of our Earth. A time had come when there were no people left who could bear children. Changing Woman lived on her own, but, as the Sun rose one day, a ray landed between her legs and entered into her, causing her to begin menstruation and eventually to become pregnant. She gave birth to twin sons, who made the world hospitable again. Then Changing Woman rubbed skin from her breasts to create the original clans of the Diné, the people of the Earth's surface, as the Navajo refer to themselves.

Changing Woman has infinite capacity to generate life on Earth, and also taught the Diné about living with *hózhó* – beauty and harmony.

The changing woman

As a woman nears her day of giving birth, the Diné traditionally gather to hold a *hózhójí*, or blessingway. Michelle Pino, a Diné nurse-midwife, has participated in many ceremonies with her community.

"The expecting mother will gather with close friends and family in a *hogan*, the traditional Navajo dwelling, for a blessing ceremony," she says. "This ceremony is overseen by a medicine man or medicine woman and takes place very late at night and continues through the morning.

"Her aunties, her husband, her friends and relatives – up to about twenty people – will gather around, with the woman at the center of the circle. They will spend the night chanting and praying for her to have a safe and quick labor, and for her to be a healthy mother with a healthy child."

Diné people believe that for something to happen you have to envision it, make it in your dream – and then it happens in reality.

– *Michelle Pino, nurse-midwife, Navajo, New Mexico, USA*

Changing Woman by celebrated Navajo basket-weaving artist Elsie Stone Holiday

"All night long, blessings and prayers are spoken, with incense burning. Corn is sacred in Navajo culture, and there are offerings of corn pollen. It's a wonderful way to support women who are getting ready to give birth, but happening less and less as people are so busy."

The *hózhójí* ends with the "Twelve-Word" song, which repeats, *"Sa'ah naagh éi, Bik'eh hózhó"* – a phrase often translated as "Long life and happiness into old age", though this does not truly capture the meaning to the Diné. The words themselves are considered to be a holy entity among these people.

Old ways, new blessings

In much of the Western world, where work so often determines that we live far from friends and family, women are creating new traditions to cement new communities – and to celebrate their journey into motherhood. Modern blessingways are not the same as the sacred rituals still practised by the Navajo people, but they are becoming increasingly popular as ways for women to support each other.

Milli Hill, founder of the Positive Birth Movement, lives in Somerset with her partner and two daughters. When she was looking for a way to welcome her third child into the family, she decided to explore how the blessingway ceremony could be adapted to her life in England.

"We had a gathering of my close women friends at my home," Milli remembers. "There were about ten of us, including my midwife, my mother and my two little girls, aged three and five, who were very excited. I wanted them both to have a very positive idea of birth; I had heard only horror stories before becoming a mother."

> I felt it would be a gift to them as women to be comfortable with birth.
>
> – *Milli Hill, founder of the Positive Birth Movement*

"Everyone brought food to share and we sat in the garden, but then we got dive-bombed by wasps. So we moved into my neighbour's bell tent, which is a lovely circular space.

"I had asked everyone to bring a poem or a piece of music, so we went round the circle and heard each one; it was very moving. One friend read a poem that another friend had written for her own birth; another played music that was playing when her child was born – so there was a sense of these lovely things being passed on.

"Everyone had also brought a bead, which we threaded onto a long piece of gold elastic which we stretched around the whole circle. My partner had given my girls a bead to give to me, so his was the first one threaded on to the elastic; it made it feel as though he was holding everything together. As each bead was threaded on to the elastic, it was passed around the circle and went through each woman's hands until it eventually reached me.

"I cut the elastic and tied it into a necklace, which I put around my neck. Then each woman cut a section of the remaining elastic and threaded on one wooden bead to make a bracelet which she would wear until my baby was born – a symbol of her connection to me.

"Then I had my bump hennaed with a leaf pattern. It was beautiful! Most of my friends had to get home to their own children, but a few of us stayed up late talking, together with my partner and my neighbour's husband.

"I am wearing my necklace of beads now, and I like the idea that, when I am in labour, all those people who are important to me will be wearing theirs too."

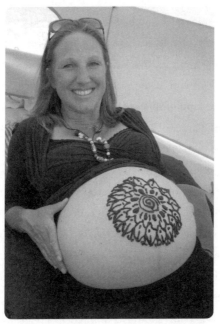

Milli at her blessingway ceremony

✳ ✳ ✳ ✳ ✳ ✳ ✳ ✳ ✳ ✳ ✳ ✳ ✳ ✳

Alive in one big mystery

All my life I was Carrie Lee, the sweet and quiet good girl, follower of rules, planner and lover of logic. Pregnancy, childbirth and motherhood helped me expand beyond that definition. In pregnancy, I could no longer deny the bigger picture. Now, I was Carrie, carrier of new life, threshold for the creative. As my soft and round belly grew, my world grew softer and rounder, more pliable, less exact. I imagine this feeling is universal among mothers, that we feel alive in the one big mystery.

Our babies swim in the waters of life, and we go searching for the same kind of spaces – places that nurture a similar fluidity, places where we can connect to ourselves, our babies and our relationships with others.

Our modern society offers most women (though not all women) birthing options and resources, but it steers us away from our ancient wisdom. This is reflected in our overly medicalized model of care, and our lack of customs that truly honor a mother's rite of passage. We hold "baby showers", which are wonderfully sweet gatherings in which the mother receives gifts for the baby, but there is something missing.

At my own baby shower, I wanted to create a space that would acknowledge the spiritual and emotional aspects of my experience, so I asked for blessings to be written down on slips of paper. I gave candles to each guest and asked that they light them when my labor began, so I could draw upon their supportive energy.

I think women ache for such spaces. And so I offer this blessing to the world's mothers:

May you recognize and embrace your divine feminine gifts. As your body transforms through pregnancy, so may your mind expand to accept the depth and power of your true self.

May you know your strength in labor and may your baby be welcomed by a mother in all her glory.

May the spirit of your family, from generations past and into the future, bless and sustain you and your baby. Just as you have nourished this new life, may you nourish your new life.

May you be born anew, with new mind, new body and new spirit so that your baby, and the world, will be blessed by your gifts.

May you allow your new story to unfold.

— Carrie Lee Ferguson, Florida, USA

5

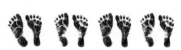

DELUGED WITH LOVE:
THE BABY SHOWER (USA)

The American tradition of the baby shower is somewhat in-
famous as a time when expecting parents receive gift after
gift from friends and family to prepare for the baby's birth. But the
tradition is also an occasion for people to show love and support for
the mother in the later months of her pregnancy.

"Wonderful friends and volunteers arrange your baby shower
for you (it's considered rather bad form to do it yourself)," explains Katy Hope, who lives in New York State with her husband
and sons, Pete and Teddy. "My first baby shower, before Pete was
born, was organized by two close friends, Liz and Robin, in Liz's
apartment in Manhattan. I was about seven months pregnant,
and we had luncheon. I'd let people know that I was expecting a
boy, and we had a cowboy theme, so there were big pots of delicious chili to share.

"We played some games with different levels of cheesiness:
measuring my belly with a piece of string to guess my circum-
ference; making anagrams of the word 'diaper'; tasting five types

of baby food to guess the flavour – all tasted the same…terrible!

"I'm in a lucky place and we already had many of the things we needed for the baby, so I didn't do the usual big gift registry. But friends gave me beautiful hand-made gifts and a lot of fun extras like little hats and socks as well as some swaddling muslins – those were useful!

"About twenty women came to the shower, including my mother and mother-in-law. I chose to make it a woman-only event, as that's when (and how) the real truth-telling starts. Liz and Robin had sent out invitation cards asking friends for their best advice, so a lot of those who couldn't come sent messages back, such as, 'Remember to take care of you' and 'There's always help if you need it – call me!' I felt very cared for.

"I also had a further 'baby warming' party with my knitting group and they knitted a baby blanket for me as well as some little knitted animals – elephants and rabbits."

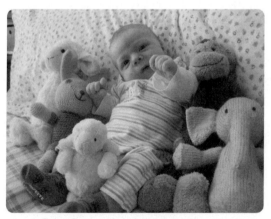

Baby Pete with hand-knit menagerie

Crossing cultures

I was caught between two cultures. My dad is Chinese and my mom is half Chinese and half Vietnamese and they live in Cambodia. Although my parents had their doubts – because in our cultural tradition it risks misfortune to celebrate the baby before he is thirty days old – my sister did give me an American-style baby shower.

Following the American tradition, we got a lot of gifts. We also played games, which tested our knowledge and got you thinking about the coming baby. For instance, my cousin bought ten bottles of baby food and people played the game of tasting them and trying to identify them. We also played a game in which smashed-up candy bars were put on a diaper, and people had to try to identify the original candy bar!

In my family's culture, people don't buy baby foods – we make a porridge of rice and take the water from the rice to feed the baby. We add one food group at a time to this broth – meat, then vegetables and so on. We don't have baby food in shops, so the baby shower was an interesting way for me to find out about what is available.

– *Kiev Martin, Maryland, USA*

A lap full of generosity

The American baby shower has equivalents around the world, though some are more focused on the mother's happiness than on building a home for the baby. On an auspicious day during the seventh month of pregnancy, Hindu women in northern India hold a *godh bharai* (गोध भराई, "fill the lap") for a mother-to-be. She is given all the gifts and love she might want at this special time. Fears for the risks she will face in childbirth seem to inspire the community to be especially generous, in case her life is cut short.

The mother is dressed in a beautiful sari and seated in a place of honour. In some families, a *puja*, an offering of devotion, is done. The guests bless the woman and place their gifts in her *godh*, or lap – clothes, sweets, jewellery or cash. Every woman who attends also whispers good wishes or reassurances into the ear of the pregnant woman. The woman's own mother or mother-in-law will have prepared all her favourite dishes. Then there is much singing and dancing to celebrate the coming of a new member of the family.

The *godh bharai* is known by other names across India: *shrimanth* in Gujarat, *shaad* in West Bengal, *seemandham* in Kerala. Among the Saraswat, it is called *baikikol*. Dr Saraswathy Ganapathy, director of projects at the Belaku Trust in Bangalore, remembers her *baikikol*, which took place far from India. "Although I was in New York for my first pregnancy and delivery and am not from the Saraswat community, my husband, who is a Saraswat, came to New York carrying all the paraphernalia for the ritual. A group of women friends, Indian and American, attended. They dressed me in a special green sari, put glass bangles on my wrists, and placed presents and fruit in my lap. We may have got a lot of things wrong, but it still felt like a very special time and the affection and concern for me and my unborn baby was wonderful to feel."

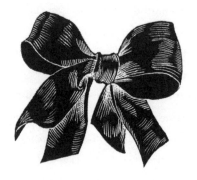

Full of health and hope

In the Merrygold Health Network of Uttar Pradesh, they host *godh bharai* ceremonies in which they fill the laps of pregnant women with a basket of nutritious foods, vitamins and information on maternal care. It is a beautiful service, full of health, happiness and hope.

By bringing pregnant women together to share stories and celebrate this joyous moment with others in their community, they also encourage women to give birth at a health facility rather than at home, so that they will have access to the tools, medicines and care that could help if a life-threatening emergency comes up during childbirth. Merrygold's *godh bharai* practice has been so effective that the government has begun work to implement it in public centres as well.

I look forward to watching as more women's laps are filled with such gifts, so that their lives have a better chance of being filled with hope.

– Priya Agrawal, executive director of Merck for Mothers, a Merrygold and White Ribbon Alliance partner

Marking the moment in history

"The baby book for my daughter was started for me by a friend and given as a gift at my baby shower," recalls Nancy Dennis, who now lives in Richmond, Virginia. "I loved it so much that I did the same for other friends.

"It has clippings from catalogues of men's and women's clothing and hairstyles, pictures of the new car models and ads showing the cost of houses and cars in the year my first daughter was born. I added captions to the clippings and collected more before (and, later, after) her birth. I then added the headline from the newspaper on the day my baby was born – there was a phone strike, so I explained in my caption to my daughter that this made it hard to get news of her birth to our family and friends. I pasted in the comic strip and the horoscope for the day. As mementos, I taped the wristbands that were used to identify both of us in the hospital – even before we had officially given her a name. And I included a copy of the doctor's and hospital bills related to her birth, so that she can compare them if and when she has children of her own.

"We received dozens of cards congratulating us on our daughter's birth, and I saved these in the book too, with notes on who the various people were, both friends and extended family. It was quite funny to see how many people chose the same card to send!

"Later, the baby book is where I saved a lock of hair from her first haircut. And through the years I added artwork or papers that she did for school, mementos from special occasions, etc.

So the book grew to be a chronicle of her life from the beginning until she took wing and flew the nest to start on her own path – so much more than a baby book."

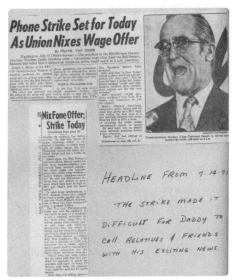

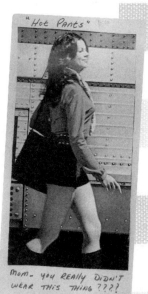

From Nancy's baby scrapbook, 1971

HEADLINE FROM 7.14.71

THE STRIKE MADE IT DIFFICULT FOR DADDY TO CALL RELATIVES & FRIENDS WITH HIS EXCITING NEWS.

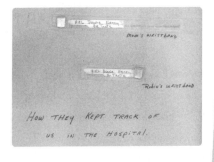

HOW THEY KEPT TRACK OF US IN THE HOSPITAL.

MOM - YOU REALLY DIDN'T WEAR THIS THING ????

6

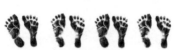

ANOINT THE BELLY:
THE OIL OF JOY (NIGERIA)

Nigeria has many tribes and dialects, and each has its own way of celebrating the birth of a child. I am an Igbo lady, married to a Yoruba man, so of course we had to struggle with differences between our tribes and cultures," says Merry Ify Obah from Ubulu Unor in Delta State, Nigeria.

"I had just finished my National Youth Service and had moved to be with my husband; soon afterwards I became pregnant with our first child. My husband and I also happen to be the first children of our parents, so there was joy all around when the news got to our family and friends.

"Right from when my baby was conceived, I anointed my belly every day and blessed her, using the anointing oil we have at church," says Merry. Inspired by Psalm 45:7, "Therefore God, your God, has set you above your companions by anointing you with the oil of joy," these oils are popular in local churches – not just during special times of joy such as pregnancy, but during any troubling situation, as a soothing agent.

"Everything to make me happy"

For Merry and her husband, Vincent, it was important to ensure a calm environment. "I played songs and read to her. I love singing and listening to music, so I always kept my iPod on my stomach for her to listen to. Now she is four years old and my daughter also loves music – always smiling, singing and dancing – so it paid off. I did this daily with the support of my husband," Merry says.

"Before the birth of my daughter, my mother came over to stay with us. She brought everything she thought I would need – and mothers know best! – from foodstuff to be eaten by pregnant women to baby items. This was the first grandchild, and in the Igbo culture the woman's mother is the one to help her. However, in Yoruba culture the father's mother helps. Thankfully, my husband agreed for my mum to be with me. He spoiled me silly. He didn't behave like most men. He did the house chores – everything and anything to have me happy."

Stretching out

Merry's husband is a wise man: a happy mother-to-be helps make for a harmonious and healthy start to parenthood. Pregnancy is a time to take special care of the expecting mother, and for the expecting mother to take time to care for herself. One of the best ways to look after mind, body and spirit is take up the practice of yoga.

Yoga has long been recognized as a safe and effective technique for making your body stronger and more supple. Yoga

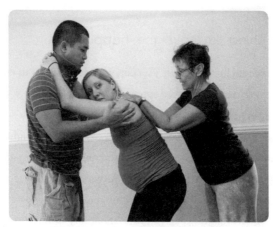

Practising relaxed labour positions

also lowers blood pressure and reduces stress, while helping you grow more aware of your own body and its amazing potential for change. Yoga classes for pregnant women also introduce mothers-to-be to each other, building a valuable support group for the years to come.

Of course, pregnancy often brings many physiological changes, often including weight gain, fluctuations in body temperature and circulation, nausea, cramps and back pain. Sometimes women experience high blood pressure and anxiety, and regular yoga practice can help. Yoga also encourages greater consciousness and control of breathing, which can prove very useful during labour and childbirth. Certain positions can help to open the pelvic region in preparation for delivery.

Lindy Roy, a specialist in yoga for pregnancy and birth, teaches Viniyoga at Yoga Māla. "This is a flowing form of yoga in which we synchronize the breath with our movements, using long out-breaths, and so it is very meditative. With the focus on long out-breaths, this can be helpful for calming the mind and emotions during labour and birth.

"If you practise yoga regularly, you begin to physically remember, so that when you are in a different zone during labour you can access your 'body memory' – and, without thinking, your body knows what to do.

"Yoga also helps pregnant women get in touch with their bodies and their babies. This is a very precious and emotionally sensitive time," says Lindy.

> Yoga can help us feel more in tune with nature and with the miracle of our journey through pregnancy.
> – Lindy Roy, yoga teacher, UK

"Many women find the skills and resources they have developed also help after the birth," she continues. "This is a period of huge change at every conceivable level, and the friendships, support and resources that women develop during their pregnancy yoga classes can be very helpful at this stage. Many women return to their pregnancy yoga classes to share their stories, maintaining their yoga friendships long after leaving their classes. And many mums return to yoga during subsequent pregnancies."

There are many ways of working with yoga in pregnancy. Lindy recommends some of these core *asanas* (yoga postures) for pregnant women:

1) *Cakravakasana*, The Cat: This is a great posture for pregnant women. One way is to move the hips

fluidly – the woman resting her knees and forearms on the ground, with her bottom in the air. This position frees up the pelvis and also encourages the baby into optimal position for birth. It can also help reposition the baby if it is breech (bottom down).

2) *Ardha Utkatasana*, Half Squat: While the full squat is not recommended in pregnancy (in case of straining the pelvic diaphragm), the half squat – rather like a seated position but without a chair – helps develop the muscle tone and strength that your thighs will need during labour and birth.

3) *Tadasana*, Standing Pose: This pose helps pregnant women to practise good posture – with chest open and lifted, broad back, weight equally balanced on the feet, legs straight and pelvis and abdomen relaxed. Good

The belly cocktail

After the birth and to help contract the uterus, the grandmothers of the land say you must heat up wine, wet cloths made of linen with the hot wine and place them on the belly. This is the perfect medication for losing the belly and getting everything back to the right place! Others mix brandy with herbs to place on the belly. As well as recuperating in bed for at least five days, for the first fifteen days you do not drink water straight from the fridge. The water should always be boiled and then cool down naturally for drinking.

– Dora Gouveia, Portugal

posture helps prevent backache and pelvic organ prolapse (both common during pregnancy and after the birth) and promotes general good health.

4) *Virabhadrasana*, The Warrior: A strong, asymmetrical standing pose – one leg is put forward with the knee bent while the back leg is kept strong and straight and the arms and chest are raised – this *asana* helps develop strength and flexibility in the legs and thighs, as well as psychological strength.

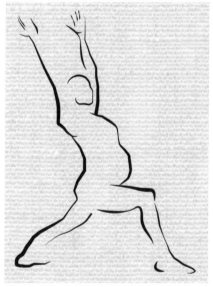

The *Virabhadrasana*

5) Rocking the hips: Rather like belly dancing, round and round, this movement often just feels right in pregnancy and birth. It helps to ease discomfort and keeps the woman upright during labour, so that gravity helps the baby to descend.

Clocking the changes

A first pregnancy is a time of unprecedented change in any woman's life. Your body, your relationships, your feelings, your dreams – all feel different, for better or for worse. These changes are profound; at times you may feel you are losing your old self in order for your new self – and your child – to be born. Keeping a week-by-week pregnancy journal can help you to take stock of these changes and their significance.

If you have a second or third pregnancy, this journal can re-mind you of how you felt and where you had reached before, as well as providing a wonderful document for your child. Some possible questions to pose to yourself:

1) How far along (week and day)?
2) How many hours of sleep each night?
3) Craving any food (or hating any)?
4) Feeling any movement?
5) Finding any positions (sitting, sleeping, etc.) or exer-cises easy/difficult?
6) State of the belly button and size of the bust?
7) Status of maternity clothes?
8) Best remedies for discomforts discovered?
9) Any changes to my body that I like?
10) Any changes I don't like?
11) Most annoying development this week?
12) Any dreams about birth and the baby?
13) Any new friends made?

14) Any new developments with my partner?

15) Any unexpected emotions?

16) Current plan for baby's birth, including who to have there?

17) Feeling sad about…?

18) Feeling happy about…?

19) Best advice received?

20) This week's new tradition or milestone?

Some women choose to share the answers to questions like these on a social network or public blog. It's up to you to decide how best to take care of yourself.

Sage suggestions

According to Tibetan thought, heavy work and frequent sex are not good for pregnant women and can harm their babies, even causing physical disabilities in the child. Yet the expecting mother should not be lazy. It is recommended that she do light housework and take walks around temples; this is believed to exercise the child, making his body supple and firm, and ensuring an easy birth for the mother. The mother should also drink water blessed by a spiritual master, to ensure her child's long life and good fortune.

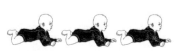

7

ROCK THE BELLY:
LENGGANG PERUT (MALAYSIA)

Seven-month ceremonies are common throughout the world, because a baby born at this time or later has a much better chance of survival. In Malaysia, the ceremony held at seven months is *lenggang perut*, which translates roughly into English as "rocking the belly".

First, a *bidan*, or midwife, examines the mother to confirm her stage of pregnancy and agrees to help with the childbirth. Once this is done, the family gathers together to say prayers for the couple and the coming baby. Seven types of flowers are mixed in water, which is then further mixed with water blessed by a recitation of the verse *Ya-Sin*, known as "the heart of the Qur'an". Finally, the juice of a lemon is stirred into this holy mixture.

The pregnant woman will then be asked to lie down on seven layers of *batik* sarongs, a traditional form of dress. Ideally, the sarongs will be seven different colours.

The *bidan* massages the mother's belly with coconut oil and places a coconut with its husk peeled off on it. The coconut soon rolls off, of course, and if it comes to a stop with its "eyes" up it is believed that the baby will be a boy. Sometimes, an egg is used instead – and, if the egg breaks open, the mother should expect a girl.

The *bidan* and older women of the family then grasp the ends of the top sarong, pulling it left and right from under the woman's hip area, gently swinging the belly and uttering prayers. They continue this until all seven sarongs have been pulled out from under her.

After the ceremony, the family and their guests will eat a special meal of *ambang*, a traditional dish of mixed rice.

Wrapped with love

The *lenggang perut* has a practical purpose: the rocking motion can help turn a baby inside the womb, to encourage a better position during gestation or for childbirth. Some believe the secret lies in relaxing the mother's body – once the mother is rocked into a state of relaxation, a slightly stronger tug to the end of the cloth on the side to which the baby should rotate often works. It can also gently massage aching abdominal and back muscles.

The Malay are not alone in using a long cloth to rock the belly. In Mexico, a *rebozo*, a colourful cloth often made from cotton and about five feet long, is used to alleviate backache, relax the mother during labour and reposition the baby too. Traditional midwives sometimes use a *rebozo* a few weeks after birth to "close up" the mother in a gentle, body-wrapping massage. When it is not being used for these purposes, the *rebozo* is worn as a shawl, or coiled and placed on the head to make it easy to carry heavy items such as a bucket of water.

Doula Stacia Smales Hill explains that the *rebozo*'s woven texture, together with its long fringe, means that the shawl can be gripped without the hands slipping – unlike with, say, a pashmina. This makes it especially suited to being a physical extension of the carer's arms. "I use the *rebozo* to hug a woman, to put my arms all the way around her so she can feel confident and safe," says Stacia. "We call it the wrap of love."

The *rebozo* is also used for the *manteada* technique, known as "sifting", in which the cloth is used to create a hammock for the mother. (Please note: proper training is essential to carry this out safely.) "If you shake a tense muscle, it helps it to relax," explains Stacia. "The same is true of the pelvic muscles, which can get very tense, so that the baby's head is pushed to the side or back. But put a woman in a position where she can relax, held by the

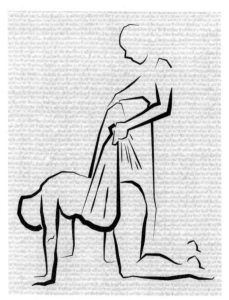

Using a *rebozo* to relieve back pain

doula or midwife in the *rebozo*, and give the muscles a bit of a shake and it can have remarkable results.

"I was working with a woman who badly wanted a vaginal birth (after a previous C-section) but the baby was facing her back and had not descended. I did the *manteada*, and we were laughing and joking," remembers Stacia. "She relaxed and, by the time I left, the baby's head had dropped down into her pelvis. She gave birth the next day."

A safe touch

The *rebozo* can also help women overcome any hesitancy around being touched, believes Stacia. In other cultures, the midwife or traditional birth attendant will be constantly massaging or rubbing the mother's arms, back, hands – but some women may feel threatened by that level of physicality, especially when they are being attended by a health worker they have never met. The *rebozo* provides an unthreatening way of being in close physical touch at the time of the most intensely physical experience of a woman's life.

Similarly, during labour, a woman may want to squat but may not have confidence in her own stability. The *rebozo* provides the extra support she needs. The shawl can be wrapped around the birth partner's waist, or the end of the bed, while the mother holds the ends and pushes down. It can also be especially useful if a woman is using a birthing pool; she can put her feet on the edge of the pool, hold the ends of the *rebozo* and push.

The *rebozo* can also make it easier to accept the father's or another birth partner's help. "Women know they are heavy and may fear their partner can't take their weight, but the *rebozo* makes that possible," says Stacia.

The seventh-month request

The birth of the first baby is regarded as woman's work in the Shona culture. The woman goes back to her parents' home when she is seven months pregnant, so that she can receive their help and advice. Her mother will prepare her for the process of birth and then look after her and the baby. The birth of a baby is a blessing and a joy!

The woman's husband gives her parents two live goats, groceries and toiletries. This denotes his formal request that his wife's parents look after her until the baby is born. The goats are slaughtered on the day of the birth and shared with the extended family. The custom is known as *kusungira*, or the "seven-month request".

This cultural tradition is still observed – with a twist – by working women in urban areas. The young couple will still present the gifts to the parents on the understanding that, when the time of birth is near, her mother will come to town to provide support.

Nowadays, the young mother's friends or fellow church members will also arrange a baby shower. These are becoming very popular in urban areas, as a way of sharing knowledge. The young mother is taught how to bathe a baby, and she learns deportment – how to walk, sit and dress; how to behave when talking; and what are suitable mannerisms, now that she is a mother.

– *Rebecca Pasipanodya, Masvingo Town, Zimbabwe*

8

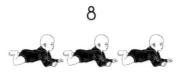

DO THIS, DON'T DO THAT:
TABOOS

It seems that everyone has advice for a pregnant woman – things that she must do, mustn't do and mustn't do except on special occasions. Some pregnancy taboos have a deep wisdom behind them, but not all make sense to us today.

What not to eat

Every culture has its own traditions about what foods and drinks should not be consumed in pregnancy. From modern Western health concerns about the risks of unpasteurized dairy products and mercury in fish, to Eastern traditions of food that have either a "heating" or a "cooling" effect on the body, rules proliferate in our attempts to keep mother and baby safe. Here is a sampling of things women are not supposed to eat while pregnant:

 ⋄ *Nsenene*, or bush crickets (Uganda): A traditional delicacy usually collected by women and children for the men of the family, *nsenene* has long been taboo for women to eat. Recently, women

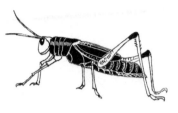

have begun to enjoy the treat – but not during pregnancy. "It is taboo for her to eat or even touch grasshoppers while pregnant, because people believe this will harm the unborn," says Samuel Senfuka, chief of the Buganda people. The worry was that the child's head would resemble a grasshopper's at birth.

⬥ Fish heads (Moldova), or else the child may be born with the head looking like a fish.

⬥ Fish with red flesh (Hawaii): This is said to risk giving the baby a red birthmark.

⬥ Eggs (Malawi): According to Lennie Kamwendo of Malawi's White Ribbon Alliance, "Some believe that, if women eat eggs in pregnancy, then the baby will be born with an oval head resembling an egg. The truth is that all babies born normally have some degree of moulding at birth, which make their heads look a little egg-shaped, but these things only last for a day or so."

⬥ Dog meat (northern China), or else the child may be born with a strong desire to bite you – making for some very uncomfortable breastfeeding. Breastfeeding can be tricky once your baby gets teeth!

⬥ Food provided by people who have neglected their moral obligations (Tibet), for fear of polluting the spirit. Overly spicy and sour food should also be avoided. Pregnant women should also stick to nourishing food and try not to overeat, despite the common saying that women are "eating for two".

✖ ✖ ✖ ✖

An environment to thrive in

When a woman gets pregnant, it is a great joy to the family, because an unknown person is going to be born. The pregnant woman is described as a fragile person and she is not allowed to do certain things. Care is taken to control her movements and activities. The environment should be conducive to thrive in.

The pregnant woman is not supposed to do strenuous activities, which will put the unborn child into danger. A responsible husband will assist his wife who is pregnant by doing some of the house chores. As the pregnancy gets to the last stage, or third trimester, an elderly woman is sent to the pregnant woman, or the pregnant woman will travel to an elderly auntie, grandmother, mother or a senior sister, so that she is looked after. At this stage, people will start teasing the pregnant woman, calling her "twin mother" or "big abdomen" or saying, "You have eaten too much".

Some cultures do not allow pregnant women to eat certain foods, like snails and hen's eggs. According to them, if the pregnant woman takes in snail, a lot of saliva will come from the mouth of the child. But, apart from that, they are made to eat an adequate, nutritious diet, foods that contain carbohydrates, protein and vitamins. They are also told to rest so that they will have enough energy to push when the baby is coming.

The Christians will go to church for prayers for safe delivery. The traditional people will also go to the herbalist or fetish priest for herbs and libation. Where there are antenatal clinics, the family or the community assists the pregnant woman to attend. Sometimes she is accompanied by a relative or a friend. This is to give emotional support to the mother and the unborn child.

– Georgina Nortey, Greater Accra, Ghana

What not to wear

It is one of the most unpredictable dangers of childbirth: an umbilical cord wrapped around the baby's neck. A skilled midwife or other health worker can save this risky situation, but the fear of this happening is reflected in taboos about mothers-to-be wearing anything around the neck.

- Necklaces, rings or hair braids (Inuit)
- A lei (Hawaii), unless it is open-ended and hangs like a scarf.
- A bra (Liberia), as this restrictive garment might cause the umbilical cord to get knotted. "So a mother-in-law might come to the woman and say, 'Take that off!'" says Gorma "Mother Dear" Cole, a well-respected nurse-midwife in Bong County.
- Revealing clothes (Tswana people, South Africa), because exposing arms, legs or cleavage may make a woman susceptible to colds. Becoming ill during pregnancy weakens the mother.

What not to close

It is remarkable how many different cultures have long-standing prohibitions against any kind of "closing" or "blocking" activities, for fear that these will translate into a blocking of the baby's passage into life, dangerously delaying birth. Women are prohibited from several activities as a result:

- Sewing or crocheting or tying any knots (Malaysia), or the umbilical cord could become twisted and tangled during birth. Mothers-to-be are discouraged from preparing outfits for their babies, as this might cause the cervix to be "stitched up" too.

✦ Standing in a doorway for too long (Liberia), "while you're talking to someone outside", says "Mother Dear" Cole, for, it is believed, "the baby's head will pop out, get a breath of air, then pop back in".

✦ Sitting in a doorway (Indonesia), which Dr Srihartati Pandi of White Ribbon Alliance says is believed might "block the path of the child and cause a difficult birth".

✦ Walking backwards over a threshold (Inuit), according to Julie Lys, a Métis nurse of Cree, Chipweyan and European heritage

Safe from the spirits

If one must attend a funeral, the Malay offer some suggestions to ensure the health of the growing baby. Before visiting the dead, a woman should recite a prayer three times, bite the *jerangau*, then rub the bitten *jerangau* at the joints. She can also protect herself by drawing a mark in lime on her abdomen before or soon after the visit.

The husband of a pregnant woman who must visit the dead need not protect himself from the spirits beforehand, but he must take precautions against contaminating the mother before he sees her. First, even before entering the house, he should take a bath – with the clothes on. After he has washed himself, the clothing must either be thrown away or scrubbed thoroughly.

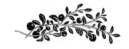

who works in the Northwest Territories, Canada. "This is because of a belief that it may cause the baby to be born in a breech position."

What not to look at

- ✧ Terrifying films (Bangladesh), as the stress might affect the baby.
- ✧ Ugly things (Philippines), in case this spoils the baby's beauty.
- ✧ A funeral (Portugal, Japan and many others), since attending a funeral exposes a woman to many spirits and feelings of negativity, which should be avoided if at all possible.
- ✧ A scary animal (First Nation peoples, Canada), in case this frightens the woman and her baby ends up looking like the animal.
- ✧ An eclipse of the Sun (Latin America); similarly, in medieval China, women were told to look away from an eclipse, and even to take their baths in spots without an eastern or southern exposure to the Sun, so as not to offend the Sun god.

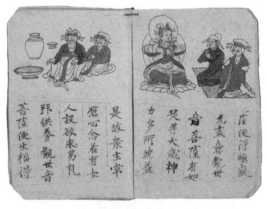

Ancient Chinese manuscript with advice for
pregnancy and childbirth

What not to do, fathers!

In our culture, we believe that, if a man sleeps with an-other woman while his wife is pregnant, this can prolong the pregnancy for extra months and also harm the unborn child. Our fore grandparents used this idea as one way to stop the husband from straying at a time when she needs his support most.

If he does commit adultery – and he is nabbed – he cannot sleep in the same bed with his wife until he has undergone a cleansing ritual.

Times are changing, so of course men are testing this, but it remains true that this is a way to ensure his com-mitment to his family and to prevent the spread of STDs and HIV.

– *Samuel Senfuka, Buganda people, Uganda*

What (else) not to do

❖ Go out at sunset (Malaysia), as pregnant women give off a special fragrance beloved of blood-sucking ghosts, who are on the prowl at this time of day. If it's necessary to go out, she should carry a sharp knife; most likely a piece of advice based on a pregnant woman's vulnerability to more common predators.

❖ Use scissors in bed (China), since cutting something (say, a piece of yarn) in this place of fertility may cut off the nourishment to the baby. On the other hand, placing a knife under your bed is good protection from evil spirits – and intruders!

Old wisdom matching the new

Pregnancy is a sensitive time when the actions and behaviours of the mother and those around her are very important, as they affect the pregnancy, birth and health of the child. Women and their partners have to conduct themselves with this awareness. It is very interesting that some of the old ideas of the Mohawk and Dene First Nation peoples are echoed by contemporary wisdom on prenatal health and wellness.

Our young pregnant women were always told by their elders to get up early in the morning, not to lie around in bed and to step out of the house straight away on rising. They should always be active, chopping kindling, working outside and inside the house, walking, walking, walking. Don't lie around on the couch watching TV. That way you will have an easy labour.

Eat just enough but not too much. And eat good foods – proteins such as good quality fish and meat, as well as berries. Don't eat too much bread or bannock or lard, or else your baby will be fat and get stuck. All this advice mirrors what we tell expecting mothers today, especially with respect to preventing gestational diabetes and macrosomia ("big baby syndrome"): take regular exercise and eat moderate portions with good proteins, limited carbs and limited fats.

After birth, our babies were always wrapped in moss bags or cradleboards. This kept them safe and warm and secure, and they learned to be very observant as they were carried everywhere and were part of everything that was going on. Hammock swings were used to soothe and settle babies to sleep. Today we know that kind of side-to-side swinging is beneficial to babies' brain development.

– *Lesley Paulette, Aboriginal midwife, Northwest Territories, Canada*

❖ Cut your hair (Moldova), should the mother want her child to have beautiful hair. If she cut someone else's hair, that person's hair would be healthy and grow quickly. Likewise, if she did any gardening, her plants would be expected to have especially lovely blooms.

❖ Take naps during the day or tickle the baby's feet (Inuit), or risk having a lazy child.

❖ Take a shower at night (Cambodia), which is said to make the baby fatter – and delivery harder.

❖ Keep quiet about the pregnancy (Moldova): Traditionally, if a mother does not speak to her friends and relatives about being pregnant, the child might be born without a voice (a form of warning that, if she doesn't share her news, they can't be helpful to her).

✳ ✳ ✳ ✳ ✳ ✳ ✳ ✳ ✳ ✳ ✳ ✳ ✳ ✳

How to stay positive

Since time immemorial, women all over the world have been deluged with advice, often contradictory, frequently doom-laden, about what to eat, how to behave and what to expect during pregnancy and childbirth. And it's understandable; we all want mother and baby to be healthy. We all want to be well-informed. But there is a downside: fear and anxiety.

Consider this: not long ago, Milli Hill decided to type "very scared of" into an internet search engine. The top four results: "labour", "flying", "giving birth" and "childbirth". So strong has the fear of childbirth become, that a term, "tocophobia", has been coined to diagnose a psychological disorder that leads some women to seek elective Caesareans rather than go through natural labour. Yet, fear itself "increases your chances of having a difficult or even traumatic experience," says Milli. "Not only can fear increase tension, which in turn makes birth more painful, but approaching birth with negative expectations can lead to a more ready acceptance of medical interventions, which usually serve to increase rather than remove any discomfort or trauma."

So how can you stay positive throughout pregnancy and birth? The best advice might be to hear the advice and then – trust your body.

> If your body has grown a baby without thought or conscious effort on your part, chances are it has a reasonably reliable plan for getting the baby out.
>
> – tellmeagoodbirthstory.com

Another great way to stay positive is to connect with other women who have had good experiences of birth – and who can tell you about it. That's why Milli, a drama therapist and doula-in-training, in 2013 started the Positive Birth Movement (positivebirthmovement.org), a grassroots organization aiming to spread positivity about childbirth via a network of free-to-access antenatal meet-up groups, linked day-to-day by social media. Within a few months of its launch, some 150 groups had been set up as far afield as New Zealand, South Africa and the USA. Women in each community gather to share their feelings and experiences – as well as tea and cake.

The movement's credo is simple: "Every woman deserves a positive birth." It doesn't have to be "natural" or "drug free". Instead, it is inspired by the rule that a woman has "the right to choose where and how she has her baby".

- ❖ Her choices are informed by reality not fear.
- ❖ She feels empowered and enriched.
- ❖ Her memories of the birth are filled with pride and warmth.

Hearing from a woman who has already gone through child-birth can also be a blessing, especially if family does not live nearby. The online group Tell Me a Good Birth Story (www.tellmeagood-birthstory.com) enables women to "find a birth buddy" who will share her story, because, as they say, "talking to a woman with a *good* birth story to tell is like having a magic key. The message 'I did it, so can you' is more powerful than you can ever imagine."

9

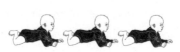

BLESSED CURD FOR A BOY...
OR A GIRL (NEPAL)

It is one of the first questions after every birth: Is it a boy or is it a girl? From the answer flows the baby's name, the clothing, the gifts, the expectations of the family – and in many cultures where males are valued more highly than females, and where physical strength is critical to prosperity or even survival, boys are more longed for than girls. Gender can be a decider of fates, and families will do all they can to influence the outcome.

Modern-day scans can reveal a baby's gender months before the birth, but what to do with this information is a big decision. Think carefully: do you want to know before the birth whether you are expecting a son or a daughter? Your relationship with your growing baby, your expectations, your hopes and dreams for your child will take colour – in more than pink or blue – from your answer. And, if your answer is yes, will you then share that information with family and friends, who will also have a hand in these expectations and aspirations?

The alternative is to wait in a state of unknowing, like that experienced by most mothers over the millennia, although it seems that every culture has tried to find some way to predict whether a girl or boy is coming.

Hoping for a son, hoping for a daughter

Samjhana Phuyal, of Nepal, remembers having mixed feelings about one traditional wedding-day ceremony in her country. "As soon as a woman is married, she is under pressure to have a child," she says. "The culture tells us that the whole purpose of marriage is to continue the family into the next generation, and that means giving birth to a son: sons not only look after their parents but they continue the male line of the family. The birth of a son is cherished in Nepalese society.

"During my marriage procession, there was a competition be-tween my family and my husband's family to see who could be the first to feed me the *mahur khuwaune* or 'blessed curd', which is a kind of yogurt made with cow's milk.

"The competition begins with the Brahmin priest uttering sa-cred chants. The curd is offered to the earth, fire and sun, and then to the bride and groom. After this ritual, the curd is di-vided equally into two parts" – one for the groom's family and one for the bride's family. Samjhana recalls that this moment was greeted with "cheering from our wedding guests and hoots from the groom's male friends and relatives".

Next, each side of the family races to be the first to feed their portion of the curd to the bride. If the groom wins the race, it is believed that the couple's first child will be a boy; if the bride's rel-atives win the race, the couple's first child will be a girl. Everyone is overjoyed, Samjhana reports, if the groom wins – both families traditionally hope for a son.

"I was unaware of this ceremony, but I could feel the excitement in the air. Before I knew what was happening, why everyone was smiling, my husband had smeared my lips and almost filled my mouth with curd. I soon learned that some of our guests then firmly believed that I would bear a son as our first child. I began to feel a little fear myself – what if it was true? I had always wanted a daughter!"

Samjhana feels that the curd race has some painful implications for mothers: traditionally, if a woman gave birth to all daughters, her husband was allowed to remarry on the pretext that his wife was not blessed by God – otherwise she would have borne a son. But she says she was lucky in that her wish for a daughter came true: "As fate would have it, and thanks be to God, I gave birth to an angelic girl the following year."

Dowsing for a boy or a girl

Expecting mothers and fathers around the world try to influence and divine the sex of their child from the time of conception.

❖ Throwing a hat in the ring (Moldova): If a couple wants to conceive a boy, they should make love at the time of the new moon, with the man wearing a hat. After making love, the man should throw his hat on the floor in a "manly gesture". However, if the couple wants a girl, they should make love at the time of the full moon, and the man should be perfectly groomed.

❖ Focusing on a gateway (Tibet): Parents who have no son may ask a spiritual master to perform a Tantric ritual using a

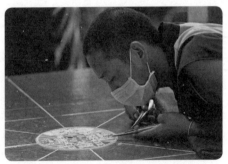

Monk creating sand *mandala*, Tibet

mandala (मण्डल), a circular symbol representing the power of the ever-changing universe that is drawn in coloured sands, in order to help them to conceive a boy.

❖ Pointing one way (Hawaii): A pointed belly and clear skin signal a baby boy is coming; a rounded belly and bad skin mean a girl – because the baby has stolen her mother's beauty!

❖ Pointing another way (Inuit): "My mother usually knew if we were having a boy or girl long before ultrasound was used," says Julie Lys, a Métis midwife in the Northwest Territories, Canada. "She would say boys are carried lower and the mother's belly sticks out more. Girls are often carried higher and lie closer to the mother's chest."

❖ Pointing yet another way (Philippines): In a ritual meant to ascertain the baby's sex, a needle is dangled from a string over the wrist of the pregnant woman. If the needle swings from side to side across her wrist, it is said she is carrying a boy, and, if it spins in a circular motion, she is expecting a girl.

The choice of nature

I've been a feminist since before I knew what the word meant. At seven years old, my dad signed me up for an all-boys baseball team because our town didn't have a team for girls. I was the only player who cried tears of joy when I hit a home run, but I was slugging it out with the boys. In college, I chose to be a women's studies major, and then went on to execute development and advocacy campaigns for some of the world's leading women's NGOs.

So I always assumed that my first child would be a girl. I would raise her to be a force of nature. She wouldn't work alongside men; men would work for her. She would be president, a hedge fund manager – you name it. Whatever the "glass ceiling" was, she'd shatter it. And all because her mother – me – would have instilled these strong feminist values in her.

And then, in 2009, I had a baby boy, Nathaniel. Four years later, his brother Joshua was born. Was my future just going to be filled with the toilet seat up and Sunday football on? I thought my dreams of raising the next great women's advocates were gone.

I couldn't have been more wrong. The first time I saw both of my boys, all I saw was endless potential, hope and love. And, from then on, I knew I was blessed to be the mother of two boys – two boys who I will guide to become men. They will be the kind of men who treat all people with respect and kindness; professionals who make the world better; husbands and fathers who won't hesitate to sign their daughters up for the boys' team, and...sons who love their mom.

– *Sara Weinstein, partner in the Weinstein Carnegie Philanthropic Group, New York, USA*

10

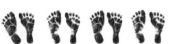

VAUVA LAATIKKO:
A BOX JUST FOR BABY (FINLAND)

In a policy that began before the Second World War, the government of Finland gives all expecting mothers what may prove to be their most practical gift: a box packed with baby clothes and other goodies. The box, which today is made of cardboard, can double as the infant's first cot. Perhaps it's no coincidence that Finland has been rated the best place in the world to be a mother.

A bountiful start

"In 1980, I was living on the island of Pelinki, and expecting my first baby, Joachim," recalls Zora King, who now lives in Scotland. "The whole atmosphere was friendly and generous; the health facilities were clean and fresh, with no waiting. I was made to feel that I was a very important person because I was creating a child. I was very well looked after.

"Along with all pregnant women in Finland, I was given a 'birth box'. It was just fabulous: inside was everything I needed to be ready for my baby's homecoming, right down to the thermometer for testing the bathwater. There were even hats and mittens, as well as the warm winter gear every baby needs in the Finnish climate – so there was little need to buy clothes. Finns always take their babies outside in their prams, even when it is as cold as minus twenty degrees Celsius, and I learned to do the same, wedging the pram in a snowdrift.

"The box was symbolic of the support that all mothers get, from advice on antenatal nutrition to how to breastfeed. And breastfeeding is very much the norm; in fact, I used to freeze some of my own milk in order to give it to mums who were having problems.

"The items in the box had no labels or branding, in contrast to the 'bounty box' I got when I eventually went back to Scotland to give birth (for passport reasons). Everything in that box was branded and it was full of leaflets on where to get more of those commercial products.

"By the time I was expecting my second child, David, I had returned to Finland. And I got a second box. David was born in hospital there, and after the dark, damp Scottish hospital where Joachim was born and where I had to fight to get a decent meal, it was a revelation – wonderful food and fresh, bright rooms, and clean nighties, dressing gowns and slippers provided for me, every day. You just had to put them in the laundry afterwards.

"The Finnish state provides a good start for all children, and I do believe that leads to a more equal society, with citizens who are well educated and well nourished."

Because all children born in the same year receive the same clothing, many Finnish parents report a sense of community with their fellow parents – and a feeling that they are in it together.

Says Zora: "This good beginning sets the tone for society's relationship with children too; children are very much included in everyday life, taken to restaurants and social gatherings where they are always the centre of attention. I think it all starts with how women are valued and supported during pregnancy and childbirth!"

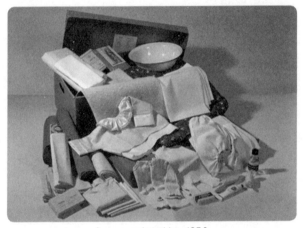

A *vauva laatikko*, 1953

Peeking inside the baby box

The goodies in Finland's baby box cover all the essentials and then some:

* A bed: the box doubles as a cot
* For bedding: a mattress, mattress cover and sheet, blanket, duvet cover, blanket and sleeping bag
* For bathing: bath thermometer, wash cloth, hooded bath towel, nail scissors, hairbrush and toothbrush

* For diapering: cloth nappy set, muslin squares and nappy cream
* For dressing in the winter: snowsuit, balaclava, insulated hat, insulated mittens and insulated booties
* For dressing in the cooler months: light hooded suit, knitted overalls, knitted hat, mittens, socks and booties
* For dressing in layers and in the warmer months: easy-to-wash bodysuits, romper suits, leggings, socks and booties
* For playing: picture book and teething toy
* For the parents: bra pads and condoms.

Mothers can choose to take a cash grant of 140 euros (£120 or $185), but more than ninety-five percent take the baby box, since it is worth a great deal more.

✳ ✳ ✳ ✳ ✳ ✳ ✳ ✳ ✳ ✳ ✳ ✳ ✳ ✳

Dear baby

On average, a woman's pregnancy lasts 283.4 days. Around her twenty-ninth week, Georgie Pope, who lives in the UK and India with her husband, the novelist Somnath Batabyal, decided to write a letter to her coming son, as a way to capture her hopes and aspirations for his future, and to prepare herself for the changes to come.

Says Georgie, "Maybe I'll share the letter with him when he's old enough to understand, or perhaps when he's old enough to enjoy it. Maybe I'll be reading some novel to him when he's twelve, or seven, or nine, and it will mention something relevant and he'll ask some question and I'll say, 'Let me read you a letter.' Maybe I'll never share the letter with him; it might be more for me than him."

204 days pregnant

Dear Robi Jo,

I've been told that, given the usual course of things, we'll meet in a little over two months. I'm looking forward to it more than I can say. Som and I will be there waiting, ready for our transformation from lovers to family. We will be three.

You and I know each other quite intimately already. My vibrations and gurgles, sleeping patterns and eating habits must be fairly well ingrained in you and I'm aware of your physical presence every waking moment.

But what about your soul? And how will we make out when we finally come face to face? Will you be a modern man who craves for chrome, steel, Apple Macs and quick solutions, amused and irritated by a quaint hippy mother, or will you grow to be wild and nomadic, a spiritual adventurer who finds me staid and conventional? Will you enjoy all the travel or crave stability? Perhaps you'll love it at first and reject it later, or insist on earning millions in an office and then take to the road again in your fifties. Maybe you will slow me down and keep me in one place after all. Will you find yourself beautiful or ordinary? Will you love yourself or yearn for something different?

I can't promise you the childhood I had, which smelt of wood shavings in Dad's workshop and of autumn leaves, tasted of homemade cake and steamed broccoli and felt like long summers on freshly cut grass. I can't promise the glorious years of camping, creative birthday parties, help with homework and endless support and attention. Will I be as good a mother as my mother? Or selfish and bored with motherhood? I'll certainly try my best. I wish you well with me.

The world is full of magical and horrifying surprises. I don't know what to make of it, and even less how it will treat you. Will it make you brittle and angry? Will you laugh and embrace its challenges? Will you be loved? Will you love?

I wish you neither riches nor penury, success nor failure. I want you to have a lot of fun and creative pleasure. I have more secret hopes, but I don't want to tell you them, in case they become weights around your tiny vulnerable baby neck.

In my mind you are – in flashes – an adult and an old man, a commuter, a schoolboy, a lover, a traveller. In two months you will be a baby again. Wrinkled, dependent and already absorbing your future. An Englishman, an Indian. Privileged. Educated parents, a clutch of languages and a mixture of influences: Christianity, Hinduism, Marxism, British Armyism, Academia, Feminism, Music, Writing. Som. Me.

What will you love and what will you reject?

Let's take it day by day. I promise to give you the space to experiment and to change, to see me for who I am and to let you in to my love for Som. We'll have fun, us three.

For now, enjoy the cosy closeness of my womb as I'm enjoying carrying you around (Delhi, London, Calcutta, Assam, Mumbai, Bristol…), and see you in just over two months, for your extraordinary and longed-for arrival.

With so much love,

Georgie (Mum)

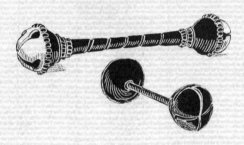

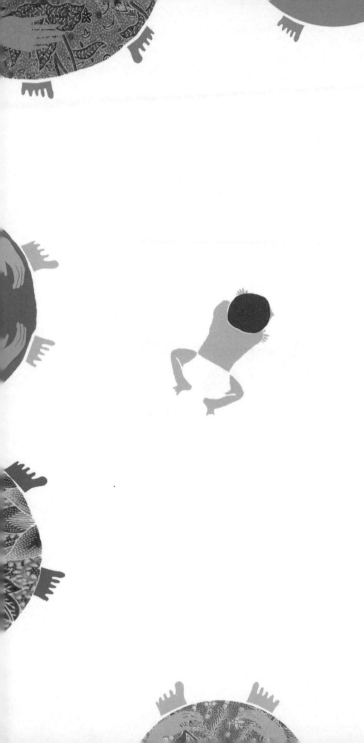

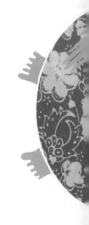

PART 2
TIME FOR BIRTH

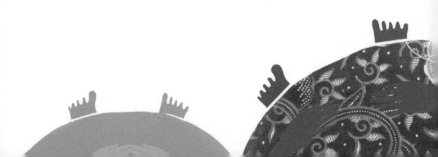

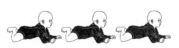

IT'S YOUR TIME, TAKE YOUR TIME
(LIBERIA)

When's the baby due?" This is the question asked of pregnant women pretty much from the start. Then, once near to or past that date – "Any sign of that baby yet?"

Yet the official "due date" is a modern, medical idea, which rarely coincides with reality. Fewer than five percent of babies are actually born on their official due date, while the average first-time mother has her baby eight days "late".

According to Milli Hill of the Positive Birth Movement, "the due date calculation is based not on ultra-modern science, but on a bungled theory about moon cycles made up by a doctor called Naegele in 1812. Unfortunately, Naegele didn't seem to be very good at arithmetic, and his dodgy old sums mean that the length of pregnancy could be as much as fifteen days longer than his 'forty weeks' target."

After forty weeks, women expecting a hospital birth can feel pressure to be induced or have their membranes "swept" – a technique meant to help get contractions started. This is because there are risks to the baby's health if pregnancy goes on too long, or if a woman's waters have broken and she has still not gone into labour. But, as many mothers and midwives will tell you, babies usually come when they are ready.

> The most important thing you can do is trust your instincts. If it doesn't feel right, don't sign!
> – *Jenn Forget, midwife*

Holding back the baby

In some parts of Africa and Asia, women have a long walk from home to the health centre. Sometimes a woman has to travel on the back of a bicycle pushed or ridden by her husband. Usually in these cases, the mother has been in labour for some time, and it is clear that things are not going smoothly. It's not uncommon for the baby to be born along the way, the cord cut by the mother and tied with a strip of fabric from her clothing. The woman will continue her journey to the health centre, where her baby is labelled "BBA", shorthand for "born before arrival".

Giving birth alone in the bush or by the side of a road in the dark is a frightening experience, which a woman will do all she can to avoid. Often, all a woman has at her defence is the power of her mind to slow the birth, in hopes that she will be able to get to a safer, more nurturing spot in time.

Liberian women say that if a baby is coming into the world too quickly – which usually means it is taking her a long time to reach the health centre – the mother can slow down her labour. "While I was still practising as a nurse and a midwife, a

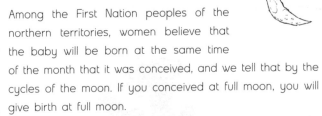

By the time of the moon

Among the First Nation peoples of the northern territories, women believe that the baby will be born at the same time of the month that it was conceived, and we tell that by the cycles of the moon. If you conceived at full moon, you will give birth at full moon.

– Julie Lys, Métis nurse, Northwest Territories, Canada

lady in labour showed up to my house one night," remembers Gorma "Mother Dear" Cole, who has been active in women's health for over thirty years and now works in the Bong County Reproductive Health Office. "I let her in and I noticed that she was unwinding three stones from her *lappa* [a colourful piece of cloth women wear as a skirt]. I asked her what the stones were for and she explained that she did not want to give birth on the side of the road while trying to get to me, so she had wrapped up the stones in her *lappa*. She believed that they would help delay the birth till she got somewhere where she could safely deliver.

"Many of the beliefs that women have are most strong out in the rural areas, where there may not be a lot of education. But women still believe it will influence their pregnancy," she says.

In *Sexual and Reproductive Health: What You Have Always Wanted to Know*, Lennie Kamwendo mentions a traditional psychological technique used by women in Malawi to slow labour. "A woman who delays going to a health centre to give birth will carry a stone on her head or her back to avoid delivering the baby on the way. I guess this is because as long as she has the stone she will have the willpower to get to the hospital before that baby comes out."

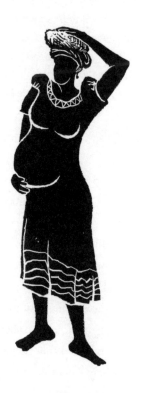

12

TAKE OFF YOUR BANGLES:
OPENING THE WAY (INDIA)

For a woman to push a child through her birth canal and out into the world is an extraordinary process, involving an almost unimaginable opening of her whole self – mind, body and spirit. All over the world, cultures harness whatever powers they can to speed and ease this opening, and to prevent its obstruction.

We've seen some of the taboos against closing things during pregnancy, against the sewing of baby clothes or the wearing of bangles or standing or sitting in doorways, all of which have been associated with a long, difficult labour around the world. It follows that, when the first contractions come, it is time to open and loosen anything and everything you can, to encourage a faster birth.

In northern states of India, traditional birth attendants will make sure that, when a woman is in labour, all the windows are opened, knots in fabric undone, locks unlocked, the woman's hair untied – even the household clay pots broken open – to encourage the opening of the mother's cervix.

In an oral history project, the Indian organization MATRIKA

collected stories from *jacc*ā (mothers) and their *dai* (birth attendant) about ways to ease delivery. For instance, Mohini from Rajasthan says that, "during labour, earthen pots with large openings are tied on top of the house. Her bangles, *bindi* and

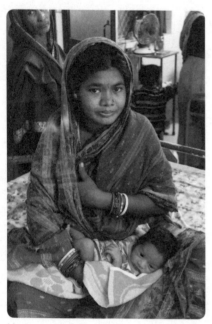
Mother with baby, India

nose ring are taken off and are offered to Bemata", a Hindu goddess who looks after the well-being of newborns. Saubatiya, a woman in Bihar state, reports: "We have a custom that the threshold is nicked, cut slightly, five times with a small knife. We open boxes, hair and all other knots."

Many of the women interviewed by MATRIKA felt there was good reason to loosen things up. "Maybe the pains are not coming because of some blockage inside. We open the blocks inside the body by opening all the outside knots. Like we take off the woman's *bindi*, bangles, hair band, locks on boxes and windows," explains Khivani from Rajasthan. And, according to a woman called Saroja in Bihar, "I was asked to come and sit in the *jacc*ā's room when my sister-in-law was in labour. She was not 'opening up'. She delivered after I came in. The *dai* said she must have been hiding something from me."

A warm welcome

Dais also follow rules of "heating" during labour, as they try to relax a mother and ease her delivery. Says Racha Kaur from Punjab, "We give a hot drink of milk and *ghee* [an aromatic clarified butter] or *ghee* and dried dates. This procedure heats and hastens delivery. It helps open the mouth of uterus."

In Rajasthan, Panna offers several options to women. "We have got a brew of *ajwain* [caraway seeds] and *laung* [cloves]. This hastens delivery. We also make a hot drink of milk, *ghee* and *jaggery* [unrefined sugar]. This procedure heats and helps in getting the pains quickly. In villages, we get *garmi ki goli* [heat-producing pills], which are given."

Sometimes warmth is applied externally. "We give hot fomentation on the lower back, by placing pieces of heated coal under the cot," a *dai* in Bihar says.

Scots unstoppering

Traditional Scottish *howdies* ("handy" women, or birth attendants) would untie any knots in a mother's clothing, uncork bottles and unlock and open the windows and doors to ensure an easy delivery.

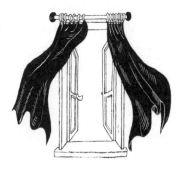

All in the mind?

In many countries, people still believe that psychological block-ages such as guilt or fear can create a physical blockage to birth, and that these feelings must also be loosened. Unfortunately for mothers in rural Mali, if a woman's labour is slow, she can be accused of being an unfaithful wife. Only when she confesses who she slept with can the baby be safely born.

MATRIKA found similar concerns in India. According to one traditional birth attendant in Bihar, "We try to find out any possible concerns of the woman, which may be why she is not opening up. Once, a woman had eloped against her parents' wishes, and it was only after her father came to the house and met her that she was able to deliver her baby."

Today, we better understand the science behind birth and the role of hormones such as oxytocin – the so-called shy hormone, which is produced in greater amounts when a woman feels safe – in opening the cervix. It is also well documented how anxiety can slow labour. "A woman's beliefs around labour, in particular her fears and concerns, have a profound impact on her ability to cope with the physical process of birth," says Maggie Howell, director of Intuition Un Ltd and the founder of Natal Hypnother-apy (www.natalhypnotherapy.co.uk). "If a woman has had many fearful thoughts about the birth, even if there is no real danger, her body responds by producing adrenaline, which will cause her to become tense and shift into a fight-or-flight state. Adrenaline suppresses the production of oxytocin, and so inhibits the body from continuing to open."

Maggie notes that "there is a growing body of clinical evidence which suggests that women who are fearful of labour are more likely to have problems and need increased medical intervention". She offers an "antidote": the use of positive visualization, where you concentrate on a mental picture of what you want to happen or feel in your body. Research has shown that visualization, especially among athletes, significantly improves "the body's ability to cope with pressure and physical performance", she says. A common visualization that women are encouraged to use during birth is that of a flower opening.

Perhaps positive visualization explains another custom shared with MATRIKA by a *dai* from Delhi: "A mound of *atta* [the wheat flour used to make *chappati* bread] is kept in a plate. The *jacc*ā takes a coin and separates it into the portions. It hastens birth." As Janet Chawla, the director of MATRIKA, explains: "Just as the *atta* is separated, one into two, so the mother and baby are, during birth, separated – the ritual being a visual analogy of the birth process."

✻ ✻ ✻ ✻ ✻ ✻ ✻ ✻ ✻ ✻ ✻ ✻ ✻ ✻ ✻

The knots in the belt

I have seen how women in labor will use a crocheted sash belt that's wrapped around the stomach for comfort and support. If the labor doesn't progress well or quickly enough, a medicine man or medicine woman may come in to untie and retie the knots in the belt, as this is thought to help to ease the birthing process.

I remember one medicine woman – a little, old granny – came into the room and began to untie and redo the knots of the sash, four at a time. The number four has sacred significance in Diné culture – because of the four seasons, and the four directions of North, South, East and West. In some of our New Mexico hospitals, sashes are available for Navajo women to hold on to and hang from during labor, as they feel that this gives them support.

– *Michelle Pino, Navajo nurse-midwife, New Mexico, USA*

13

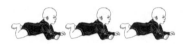

MOTHERING THE MOTHER:
THE MIDWIFE

Birth is simultaneously a time of extraordinary power and of intense vulnerability, when women may emerge triumphant – or may need the strength of others to see them through. A truly skilled birth attendant has not only the technical knowledge to save a mother's life in an emergency, but also the love and compassion that will ease her through a safe delivery. Two American midwives – who are friends as well as colleagues – share their perspective.

To be petted and comforted

Jody Lori spent time as a midwife in Bong County, Liberia. There, she helped to build maternity waiting homes – buildings where women stay before childbirth, so that they are in close proximity to trained carers and medical supplies when they go into labour.

"In the villages, traditional birth attendants or traditional midwives usually attend deliveries," Jody remembers, "and women often first go to a traditional midwife when they realize they are pregnant. One of the things the women say is that they like to be 'petted' by a midwife, because it makes them feel comforted.

"The communities with maternity waiting homes asked that they be run by a traditional midwife so that these women could remain involved and be a source of comfort for mothers. These attendants provide a support that women feel they don't always get from a trained, certified midwife. Often the traditional midwife is from the same community the mother is from, and will act like a doula."

The midwife will "mother" the mother, rub her back, help her feel less vulnerable.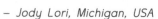
– Jody Lori, Michigan, USA

"The traditional midwife understands the process of birth, and so she can be an advocate on behalf of the mother," says Jody. "Ideally, the certified midwife and traditional midwife work together to make the birth as comfortable as possible."

To be a champion

That sentiment is shared by Annie Clarke, who began her career as a nurse in Sacramento, California, in the 1970s. A new mother herself – she adopted one child and gave birth to another – she was then working in the intensive-care nursery of her hospital. But she quickly saw the infants who were not in intensive care were also kept apart from their mothers. "At that time, they took your newborn and put it in a nursery, only bringing it out at four-hour intervals, which was not good for breastfeeding. And women gave birth on delivery tables in lithotomy position [lying on their back with their knees bent and their feet in stirrups]. It was really awful," Annie says.

She decided to attend a meeting for families who wanted to change hospital childbirth practices. "Over one hundred people were there," she remembers. "Then I was invited to my first home birth, by a family who wanted someone there with professional expertise – just in case. The mom and baby were fine. As a gift, they gave me a portable oxygen tank and said, 'You'll be needing this a lot more!' Those were prophetic words.

"I attended many more births, in the city, in the mountains, in a migrant worker's cabin, in the homes of doctors and lawyers, in a school bus. Towards the end of that time I was attending about ten births a month.

"There was no midwifery education program in the state of California at the time, and no means for a licensed registered nurse to attend home births. I stood to lose my license if anything went wrong. But women were very determined to avoid hospital and, if there was no other choice, would give birth at home without a qualified attendant or with no attendant at all. The women and their husbands and families were very happy and very relieved that I was willing to attend them."

The right to birth choices is both a woman's right and a human right.

– Annie Clarke, nurse-midwife, California, USA

"I had apprenticed for six months with a nurse-midwife trained in England who was attending home births in the US (also on the quiet). I told some obstetricians I knew about the emergency equipment and supplies I carried with me – the portable oxygen tank, masks for mother and baby, a resuscitator bag, drugs for management of postpartum hemorrhage, and so on. Some supportive obstetricians provided 'back-up' in case of emergency. Their patients planning home births would see them for antenatal care and I could call to consult with them."

But not all doctors were supportive. "There were obstetricians who would discharge a patient from their care if they found out she was planning a home birth," Annie says. "The woman

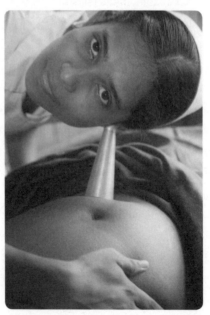

Midwife listening for the baby's
heartbeat

A midwife's top ten tips for mothers-to-be

What makes a great birth experience?

1) Getting support from a loving partner and family

2) Having a sense of being in control, even when you don't know what's going to happen

3) Being seen for who you are; being heard and listened to

4) Being encouraged to go on at those moments when you may doubt yourself

5) Attending yoga and active birth classes, to gain confidence in your body's ability to give birth

6) Getting access to a birthing pool

7) Staying active during birth – moving into different positions and remaining engaged with the process

8) Remaining calm no matter what situations may crop up

9) Being treated always with kindness

10) Having a confident yet gentle midwife who doesn't stress you out

– *Eleanor Copp, nurse-midwife, Somerset, UK*

would get antenatal care and just not tell them about their plans. Thankfully, transfers to hospital were rare. In those early days, there were six cases out of 152 women, and only two required Caesarean sections."

The mother is in charge

"The 'rules' gave the power to the hospital staff, not to the women. But, in a woman's home, she is the one in charge," says Annie.

"The birth attendant is *invited* into her home. The mother wears what she wants to wear – or even nothing at all. She has the family and friends with her of her choosing; sometimes her other children too. She can move about freely, go outside if she wishes, labor and even deliver in water, keep her baby right next to her without interruption. The bonding that occurs between mother and baby and other family members is much stronger as a result. The most important emotional or human element for birth is loving, caring support.

"I consider it a privilege to attend births no matter where they are, to serve women, newborns and their families. I am not unique in that respect, but still, I feel truly blessed!"

Holding her hand

The vice-president of global outreach for the American College of Nurse Midwives, Suzanne Stalls, has worked as a midwife in New Mexico for more than twenty years. She has assisted in many births, including her daughter-in-law's. Suzanne recalls:

"My daughter-in-law wanted her first birth to be at home, and asked me to be there for support along with her husband, my son. But after her waters broke she developed a fever and we had to transfer her to the hospital."

There, she was given Pitocin, a synthetic form of the hormone oxytocin, which helps to speed childbirth. "Soon she began active labor and had that moment of panic some women experience when they realize what is about to happen. She said to me, 'I don't know if I can do this.'

"But she lifted herself through that moment. She went to sit in a rocking chair, and was rocking back and forth with each contraction, using her breath to work through it. She insisted on having a person hold each hand and each foot. If we weren't right on it at the right time, she demanded, 'Hold my hand! Hold my foot!' But at the peak of each contraction, she would smile."

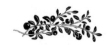

There came to my assistance
Mary fair and Brigid
As Anna bore Mary
As Mary bore Christ
As Eile bore John the Baptist
Without flaw in him
Aid you me in my unbearing
Aid me, oh Brigid

– *Gaelic prayer to Brigid, the Celtic goddess of fertility*

Belief enough for both of us

I love giving birth. I have been so, so blessed to have my babies at home, because hospitals frighten me. Home to me feels safe. It's not for everyone; if someone wants a C-section or an epidural, let them have it. But I felt I was in control of the whole experience – and that's what's made me so evangelical about it.

All my babies were delivered by midwife Pam Wild. With Chester, my last, I had done the school run, made dinner, put the kids to bed – and was having incredible "rushes" [contractions]. Pam came over ready to stay the night, and she said to me (everything was a bit slow): "I'm going to the supermarket to get a few things. You stay on the sofa, get 'jiggy' with it, it might bring it on." Hilarious! We did lots of laughing in labour!

I needed to sleep but I woke up at four in the morning with the rushes. My husband is not good at that time of night, so I tiptoed down the corridor to where Pam was sleeping and said, "Pam, I can't sleep. Can I get into bed with you?" So I did. We chatted and then we got up and walked around. I love Pam; she made me feel so beautiful and strong and, most importantly, safe.

Later, I got into the birthing pool, and my five-year-old came to join us. She said, "Mummy, just look at your boobies! They're enormous! And all floaty in the water!" By that time, it was all quite intense, an incredible harnessing of energy I didn't know I had. Of course it hurts – it is like delivering a football – but having my daughter there helped me to be brave. I didn't want her to see me screaming; I didn't want that to be what she imagined when she thought about birth. So I mooed! Then I saw my little girl take off her jumper, and next

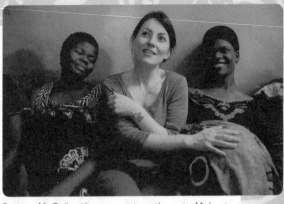

Davina McCall with pregnant mothers in Malawi

her dress, and I could see she wanted to get in the birthing pool with me. At the same time, I saw Pam getting out her sieve and I thought, *This is probably not a good idea.* So I said to my little girl, "Now I'm going to make some quite loud mooing noises." She replied, "Hmm, I'm going to watch TV. Call me when the baby's here."

Caroline Flint was the midwife with Pam for my first birth. It was thirty-six hours; we were on our knees, and it really made a difference having her there. At one point, Caroline said to me, "It could be twenty-four hours more." I just didn't think I could do it. "Twenty-four hours! I can't do it! Maybe I should have a C-section!" But Caroline held my hand and looked me straight in the eyes and said, "Yes, you *can* do it," and I said, "Okay." I didn't believe in myself, but she believed in me enough for both of us.

Midwives rock. The power of a woman helping another is without parallel. I'm so pleased that I was helped to do it the way I did. I've read Ina May Gaskin's *Spiritual Midwifery* three times; what an amazing woman. She helped me a lot.

When my babies were born, I felt like I was the lion king. I wanted to go to pride rock, lift my baby up and roar. Nothing else has ever made me feel like that!

– *Davina McCall, TV presenter for* Big Brother *&* Long Lost Family

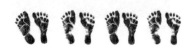

14

THE CIRCLE OF LABOUR
(MAURITANIA)

American nurse Theresa Shaver served as a midwife in Mauritania from 1980 to 1983, having moved to the country to work with the nomadic Moor people when she was twenty-five years old. Most of the Moor people are Sunni Muslims, but they also have deep traditions linked to their Berber and Beja identity. Still, the strict observance of Islam means that women are segregated from men.

The differences from Theresa's life in the USA did not end there. "My training and experience was 'high tech', but the community had no electricity or running water," she says. "I was the first *faranje* [white foreigner] to work there, and initially the children were terrified by my color; they thought I was a ghost. Everyone assumed I would leave at the first sandstorm, and were sorry for me that I was not yet married.

"When the people were away on their seasonal travels with their camels and a woman went into labor, the husband would come to the village clinic to find me, and put me on a camel or donkey to take me into the desert to help his wife.

"The clinic had a wonderful midwife called Luana who was my guide and mentor. I was able to teach her a simple form of resuscitation that you can do if the baby has inhaled meconium or can't breathe after a long labor, and I showed her how to boil and sterilize a needle. But she taught me many invaluable things. For instance, we only had a few needles, and she showed me how to sharpen them on a stone so that we could reuse them. Though I accompanied her everywhere, it took a while for the women to accept me."

They sing out so all can hear

"On one occasion, Luana and I went to assist three women who were giving birth at the same time in a hut," Theresa remembers. "The women were distressed and crying, but Luana walked in and calmed it all down. She put me in charge of one of the births. I had to be covered over completely in a large cloth – I think it is to protect the woman's modesty. It was a strange situation for me, because I was between the woman's legs, but as if I were in a tent, with only the light of a paraffin lamp to see by. The birth went well, and word got out that the *faranje* midwife was okay.

"Slavery still goes on in some places and there is a harsh class system, but during childbirth it doesn't matter what class you are – women simply surround and encircle the birthing woman."

> Sisters, mothers, and friends are with the woman day and night, humming and singing from the circle.
>
> *– Theresa Shaver, founder, White Ribbon Alliance*

"Despite aspects of the culture that oppress women, during birth they are very strong and united, with their own special power. And, when the baby comes, they all raise their voices and sing out that the child is born so that all can hear."

Surviving with support

Theresa knows how very precious the support of others can be during a difficult labour. "I have seen how much men will do to save the lives of women. One man came on his camel to the village, and said his wife was dying in childbirth. I started out following him in a car, but it broke down, so I continued on a donkey, following his camel. We journeyed all night and in the morning arrived in a small nomadic encampment. His wife was on the verge of death, and I tried to do what I could; she was very dehydrated so I gave her goat's milk with sugar, but she was almost comatose. I told the husband she needed to be taken to the district hospital.

"He had five wives but he desperately cared for her, so he went out again on his camel to get a vehicle that could take her to hospital. That took another whole day and night, and then a vehicle came over the dunes. We put her in it, with her husband, and I was relieved when news came that she had made it. Tragically, however, her baby died."

Squat and push

In the former Soviet republic of Tajikistan, I found that women were treated kindly and respectfully, but the Soviet way of birth was not woman-friendly. During labor, women were placed on delivery tables with their legs up in stirrups.

After some work, I convinced the midwives to allow the birthing women to squat. It was a great moment when one of the midwives squatted behind a woman during her labor, to give her support while she was pushing.

Nothing succeeds like success, and, once the midwives saw how this could speed a labor when a woman was not making progress, they adopted it widely. That midwife became a proselytizer for squatting!

– *Annie Clarke, nurse-midwife, California, USA*

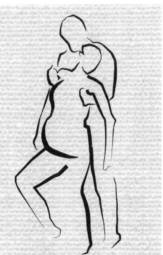

Supporting a woman during labour

Theresa founded White Ribbon Alliance for Safe Mother-hood in 2002. She says, "We do so underestimate the strength of women around the world. We often talk of them being 'poor' and victimized, but their communal spirit is incredible. They survive things that you and I would not, and I do believe it is because of the extraordinary, collective support they give each other.

"When you stand in that circle surrounding the mother, you feel the power of it. Those women are all fighting for the sur-vival of the mother. They've been there, and they are *willing* the woman to come through. I believe it really does keep the mothers alive."

Widening the circle

"Doula" is a relatively new word for an ancient role: a woman who supports other women practically and emotionally through pregnancy and beyond. Doulas form part of a team with the woman's chosen midwife, doctor and partner, filling any gaps in care, but their role is deliberately not a medical one.

According to Rebecca Schiller, the co-chair of the charity Birth-rights (birthrights.org.uk), which advocates for human rights dur-ing pregnancy and childbirth, some doulas focus their energies on the new family, cooking nutritious meals, making tea, doing light household tasks and giving guidance on breastfeeding; the involvement of a doula appears to increase breastfeeding rates. "Often the most crucial part of the role is simply being there to listen to hopes and fears, without giving unasked-for advice – being an unbiased sounding board," says Rebecca.

"I became a doula after hiring one during my first pregnancy.

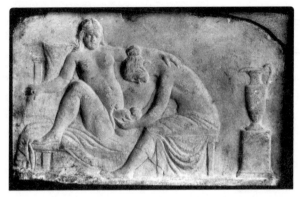

Ancient Roman carving of midwife with mother

Most of my friends hadn't felt as powerful and safe as I had when they were pregnant, and I felt called to help ensure more women had access to the support they need during this time.

"So many women today haven't held a baby until they hold their own, have no experience of childbirth or breastfeeding and feel frightened by negative media stories around birth and new parenthood. By being a doula, I feel I am helping to fill this gap. I love helping new families build their confidence and work out what is right for them.

"There is growing evidence that the support of a doula not only increases women's satisfaction with their birth experiences and decreases the duration of labour but also reduces the need for pain relief or medical intervention.

"Being a doula has made me passionate about ensuring all women have access to respectful care during pregnancy and birth and that their rights are respected." ✖ ✖ ✖ ✖

Her own song

I got a call one night from the nurse at the hospital, asking me to come in as soon as possible. A Navajo woman had arrived, close to giving birth. When I got to the delivery room, there she was with her mother, her grandmother and three or four sisters or cousins. She was sitting upright, in active labor, and her women relatives were in a ring around the bed. It was such a beautiful sight; the women's clothes were very colorful, their long lustrous hair was shining in the low light, and I will always remember the grandmother's hair, shot through with grey.

Every time the woman had a contraction she sang the same song, over and over again – it was without words and to my untrained ear sounded like "Ay yai yai yai". Women in Navajo culture are traditionally told they cannot cry out or scream in childbirth – perhaps for fear of attracting predators or enemies. This was not a scream, but a way for her to control her breath through her contractions; the repetition helped to keep her centered.

The relatives around her provided a great cushion of love and support. It was just gorgeous. The symbolism of the circle played out on so many levels – the circle of her vagina, of the baby's head, of her family surrounding her. During childbirth, we find many amazing ways to deal with stress and pain.

She sang her way through the birth, and produced a fabulous, healthy daughter with a wonderful shock of black hair.

– *Suzanne Stalls, nurse-midwife, New Mexico, USA*

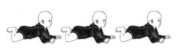

15

FATHER'S DAY TOO
(QUECHUA)

Men at the birth? It is taboo in some cultures, pretty much mandatory in others. So what can a new father do to make sure that all goes well with the birth if he does choose to be there?

Love is the key. More than at any other time, a woman giving birth needs to feel loved, safe, secure, relaxed, comfortable and protected. The father, together with her other supporters, has a vital role to play.

The birth hormone oxytocin – sometimes called the "shy hormone" given how much its production depends on a sense of safety and privacy – is also known as the "hormone of love". A partner's romantic skills in creating a warm atmosphere help to foster it. And, just as with those romantic moments, worries, interruptions and rushing will spoil the atmosphere.

This is a time for the woman's partner to really be there for her, protecting her, even speaking as her advocate, if needed. But a word of caution: men often feel they have to "do something" when the going gets tough. Normal labour and birth may look quite alarming; a woman giving birth is likely to breathe hard, cry out, moan and rock herself. Resist the urge to intervene or take over.

However, a lesson may be learned from the Quechua, an indigenous people of the Andes. Among the Quechua, the father is involved directly in childbirth. Indeed, the man is so involved that traditional depictions of labour seem to show *both* parents giving birth.

A birthing scene from Sarhua, Peru, shows a woman sitting on her husband's lap and pulling a rope. The midwife kneels in front of them. People who came to visit during the labour would be served *chicha* (corn beer) from a pot tended by a female relative. Elsewhere in the house, a shaman attempts to foresee the child's future – a gourd would be used while chanting prayers.

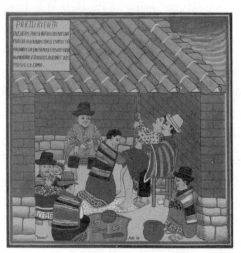

Tapestry from Sarhua, Peru

A rope to hold onto

During labour, First Nations women traditionally used a rope, sometimes made from moose hide, hung from an overhead beam in the cabin or tent, or attached to a pole in the ground or even the bed frame. The mother stood or kneeled or squatted and pulled on that when she had her labour contractions. Women helped women, but sometimes men had to help too, especially in the bush when a family was travelling alone and there was no one else to help. Her husband had to know what to do, to make a shelter for her and provide warmth and care for the mother and newborn until they could continue on.

– Lesley Paulette, Aboriginal midwife, Canada

And the father's collaborative role does not end with delivery. Babies and small children among the Quechua are often seen wearing a *chullo*, a small hat made from sheep or alpaca wool with flaps to cover (and warm) the ears. A child's first *chullo* is received at birth. That *chullo* is traditionally hand-knitted by the baby's father, and offered as a gift to the newborn. If a man cannot knit, it is his responsibility to find a close male friend who can do the job for him!

An anchor through it all

Each birth marks not only the arrival of a child, but the birth of a new mother and a new father too. So the bond between the parents during labour and delivery is important – and oxytocin, which is called the hormone of love because it is produced during sex, most likely plays a big role.

"A young woman came to live in our community from Mexico from about the age of sixteen," recalls New Mexico resident Suzanne Stalls, vice-president of the American College of Nurse Midwives. "When she went into labor she had no one with her except for her husband. A lively, funny person by nature, she walked and walked around the room quite seriously, until she was ready to give birth. With every contraction she would put her

An apocryphal tale

A woman was trying to give birth, and her husband was in the room, doing his best to be helpful but, in his nervousness, making it hard for the mother to focus. Her labour stopped progressing.

The midwife, picking up on the husband's anxiety, kindly suggested that he take the dog out for a walk in the park. He readily agreed and, as soon as he had left, the woman was able to reach the zone of intense concentration she needed in order to give birth. Before her husband returned, the baby was born.

He was delighted by the news. "Thanks for suggesting I take your dog for a walk! I've left it in the garden," he said to the midwife.

She replied, "It's not my dog. I thought it was yours."

To which he said, "We don't have a dog."

"Nor do I."

They looked outside together but the dog had gone home.

– Kathy Herschderfer, midwife, Netherlands

arms around her husband, hugging him so tightly, and she would murmur endearments in his ear: '*Mi querido, mi amor, mi vida*' ('My dear, my love, my life').

"It was such an incredible display of love that I almost felt as if I should leave the room, almost as if they were making love. He was clearly her anchor; she needed him and he was entirely there for her, as absorbed in her as she was in him.

"She soon pushed out the baby, who was incredibly sweet, and then she was back to her funny, jokey self. But I had seen her deep capacity for love and affection, and the strength of the bond between her and her husband. I felt I had participated in the forging of a family."

When the emotional side of childbirth goes well between a mother and her partner – the mother feeling completely supported and admired for her strength and power – it helps to create a lasting bond for their future.

"You're here"

"When we arrived at the birthing centre at eleven fifteen and the midwife said to me, 'You will deliver the baby,' I thought she was joking," remembers Reg Matheson of Somerset, UK. "*How sweet*, I said to myself, *she is really trying to involve me*. But, when it came time for the birth, the midwife was not even in view!

"At midday, my wife, Misty, breathed our baby out into the world. I was there in the water as she pushed our baby out, and I caught her in my hands. This wonderful, beautiful creation of love was still asleep! I lifted our daughter, Dusty Rose, out of the water and passed her into Misty's arms. It was the most incredible moment, and a fantastic privilege.

"We woke up Dusty Rose and Misty held her close to her chest," Reg says. "After the first feed, I held my daughter tight to me and just said, 'You're here, Dusty Rose, you're here.' She had the steadiest gaze and the longest eyelashes I have ever seen. I couldn't wait to bring Indiana, our seventeen-month-old son, into the loving, peaceful space that Dusty Rose had brought with her, when she came into this world."

Board and lodging

Among the Navajo and other indigenous peoples of North America, a cradleboard was used to carry and protect the baby on the mother's back, or in a spot near her work, until the baby could walk. The board was usually made by the baby's father, a symbol of the shared roles of both parents in raising the newborn.

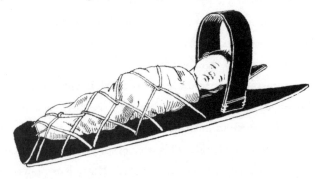

Ripping yarn

For parents and families, there is no more important and happier day than the birth of the baby and, in some rural and remote areas of Serbia, people still believe that life without children does not have a purpose and it is believed to be a punishment.

In Serbia, it is not common for the father to be present during birth. Until recently, hospitals were very strict in their attempt to protect the new mother and baby from infections and visitors, and even fathers were not allowed to visit. Although fathers are now allowed to share this precious moment with their partner, the majority still opt not to be there.

Instead, a father celebrates the news among family and friends with music, loud singing and unlimited amounts of *rakija*, a Serbian spirit typically made from plums. Neighbours, friends and family visit the new father to congratulate him, when they rip the father's shirt, wishing him and his family good health and long life.

It is said that in the old times it was not rare for babies to be born out in the field or in the woods, and the family needed something to warm the baby – hence, the ripping of the father's shirt. But they would never use a piece of women's clothing for this.

Now this is seen as a way of expressing happiness: the new father is proud, the family is expanding and his own clothes are not enough for him.

– *Jelena Vulinovic-Zlatan, London, UK*

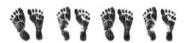

16

BEFORE THE LAST PUSH: BUILDING A SACRED *CHAKRA* (ACHUAR)

Deep in the Amazon rainforest live the Achuar people, a nation of warriors with a long history of defending their ancestral lands," explains Robin Fink, the programme director of Jungle Mamas, a project of the Pachamama Alliance that trains women about prenatal care. "Families live largely off what they are able to hunt and cultivate in their garden, called a *chakra*. The *chakra* is a sacred garden space where each Achuar woman grows manioc root, the primary source of nutrients for her family. Plantains, taro, fruit trees, sweet potatoes, herbs and medicinal plants are also grown there.

"Early each morning, Achuar women wake up to work in the *chakra*, to clear it of weeds. They use a machete to cut down trees and large shrubs, requiring great strength. Women will sing *anents*, or chants, as they work, calling upon the blessings of the female spirit who looks over the forest and the *chakra*. Singing to this goddess ensures the woman's *chakra* will produce copious quantities of manioc and taro, securing her family's well-being.

This day-to-day work in the *chakra* makes Achuar women feel very connected to and protective of the forest.

"Birth in Achuar culture is completely sacred, and the only individuals present during the process are the mother and her baby. Historically, women give birth alone in the quiet and solitary realm of their *chakra*."

The secret garden

Robin continues: "A woman will prepare the birth place within the garden by creating a support structure made out of two palm tree posts stuck into the ground with a further post suspended horizontally between them. Underneath this structure, she will place banana leaves, upon which she will give birth. During labour, the mother will crouch and hold on to the posts for support.

"During the birth, an Achuar woman will not let out cries of pain, largely due to the belief that the forest goddess will hear the

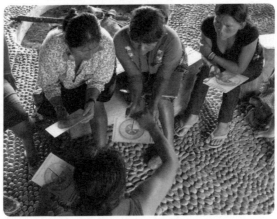

Achuar women learning about safe birth

mother's screaming and curse the child with bad temperament throughout life."

> To deliver peacefully in the *chakra* is to welcome the new being into a life of peace and tranquillity.
> – *Robin Fink, Quito, Ecuador*

"It is also a way for an Achuar woman to demonstrate and connect to her extreme strength and power, known as *kakaram*," Robin says.

She notes that Achuar women typically have between two and twelve children, and may not have enough time between pregnancies to recuperate fully. In addition, their diets have changed significantly in recent decades as their territories have been encroached upon by airstrips and other development. "Anaemia is common, which means blood loss is especially dangerous," says Robin. Haemorrhage after childbirth is the most common cause of death.

In 2007, a visiting midwife from the USA, Margaret Love, joined forces with a young indigenous leader, Narcisa Mashienta, to find ways to ensure safe yet culturally respectful birth for Achuar women. Together, they founded the Jungle Mamas programme – known in the Achuar language as *Ikiama Nukuri*, meaning "mothers as protectors of the forest".

✳ ✳ ✳ ✳

A place of peace

Women need peace and a safe place to give birth.

Natural childbirth guru Dr Michel Odent argues that we are mammals, and our human bodies already have the necessary wisdom to create and give birth to a child, despite what we might know or think. He uses the story of Adam and Eve to illustrate the risks of intellectual knowledge (via the forbidden fruit), which condemned women to suffer in labour.

While some mammals, such as dolphins and elephants, will be protected by other members of their group during labour, most just get on with it, according to Maggie Howell, the founder of Natal Hypnotherapy. If we can reconnect with the part of our brain that knows instinctively what to do, childbirth – while always a momentous and challenging experience – can also be truly wonderful.

Above all, says Maggie, "A mammal will not give birth if she feels that she is in danger, threatened, observed or disturbed. Somehow, a powerful response in her body kicks in to enable her to stop or slow down the labour until she can get somewhere safe and allow the birthing to continue."

Indeed, many midwives report that women who have been making good progress at home may get into hospital after a stressful journey and find on admission that they are no more dilated than when they left home.

Finding your safe spot

The Hadza people of northern Tanzania survive as hunter-gatherers, as their ancestors have done for thousands of years. They make their home in a region where the massive baobab tree grows. A source of nourishment, firewood and shelter, it is known as the "tree of life".

One version of the Hadza creation myth, collected in the 1960s by Peter Enderlein, says that Tsikaio, the wife of the ancestor Hohole, went to live in a baobab tree for six days, at the end of which she gave birth to a son, Konzere. The Hadza people are the descendants of Konzere and Tsikaio. Some Hadza women still use the inside of a hollowed-out baobab tree as a safe and secluded space to give birth, staying there to rest after the baby is born.

A calm, quiet space, where we can relax, feel safe and uninterrupted, is a huge help to the work our bodies have to do.

Messing with the matriarchy

Pregnant and excited, I met my husband's eldest sister for the first time while I was lying on a hospital bed in Los Angeles. She was expecting to be let into the delivery room, but, in my Western way, I didn't want any of it. I wanted to share the moment with only my husband, and I shunned my sister-in-law like an outcast. It took me years to realize how hurtful I had been to a woman who saw her place as the eldest daughter of a tough Persian matriarch who had raised seven children on the fumes of poverty.

My labor did not go well. Unfamiliar with the pain of birthing and having free and unfettered access to an epidural, I lost my maternal instincts and became incapable of pushing properly. My baby was stuck in the birth canal and I was unable to push her out. After hours of pushing and being prodded by every available nurse and eventually physician in the ward, my doctor decided I would have to have a suction cup inserted into my body to pull out the baby by the head. Exhausted, I barely understood the perils. My husband looked petrified.

Thankfully, a beautiful baby girl came out – with a head shaped like a cone. I remember the doctor cleaning her up and putting a knitted cap on her head to keep her warm, and the little pink beanie sticking up like a traffic cone. My husband was crying and I was still in shock. But my little girl was adorable.

I work now for the Fistula Foundation, and I have come to learn about obstetric fistula, where a hole is created between the wall of the vagina and the rectum or bladder during prolonged labor. I think a lot these days about what might have happened to me, or my now brilliant teenaged daughter, if we had not been so lucky.

– *Maryam Zar, California, USA*

The ten best places to become a mother

Becoming a parent is a very subjective experience, full of hopes and fears, guided by customs and celebrations, all over the world. The not-for-profit organization Save the Children has developed a more objective yardstick to measure the best and worst places in the world to be a mother, based on analysis of maternal health, children's well-being, educational attainment, economic status and women's political involvement. They publish their findings each year in the *State of the World's Mothers* report.

The top ten

1) Finland, home of the *vauva laatikko (baby box)*

2) Sweden, with a *föräldraledighet* (parental leave) system that gives parents up to 480 days of combined leave per child – 420 of them paid at eighty percent of salary (up to 910 kronor a day); if the parents split the days equally between them (240 days each), they receive a bonus!

3) Norway, where, according to Cathrine Streeval who lives in Oslo, women are provided with "rigorous breastfeeding training in the hospital after the birth, with a follow-up six weeks afterwards. Women breastfeed everywhere and no one looks on it as inappropriate."

4) Iceland

5) Netherlands, where every mother is entitled to eight days of care in her own home after the birth

6) Denmark

7) Spain, where mothers are entitled to a *reducción de jornada*, a shorter work day or work week, when they have a child eight years old or younger

8) Belgium

9) Germany, with its strong *hebamme* (nurse-midwife) service that provides home visits before the baby's birth and care treatments including acupuncture

10) Australia

The bottom ten

167) Côte d'Ivoire

168) Chad

169) Nigeria, where the government has recently backed the rights of women in childbirth by adopting the White Ribbon Alliance's "Charter for Respectful Care"

170) Gambia

171) Central African Republic

172) Niger

173) Mali

174) Sierra Leone

175) Somalia, where babies have the highest risk of dying on their birth day

176) Democratic Republic of Congo, where one in twenty-four women die during childbirth

17

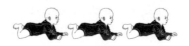

FIRST SIGHT:
BETWEEN SHOCK AND LOVE

For such a long time, you grow this invisible being who begins to move and jab and kick," says Catherine Hester, a mother of two in the UK. "And, on rare occasions, you can hear this deep heart beat inside your tummy that belongs to someone else, someone magical and incredible. Oh, how I loved that sound! Then one day it all happened."

Catherine's first child, Oscar, was born in hospital. "With Oscar, there was pain and sometimes moments of panic. But then, when I thought I couldn't bear it and it would never end, this incredible person was there: naked, warm, screaming and perfect! Oscar was so heart-stoppingly beautiful, as if he had been crafted by an angel just for me. After decades of holding and loving so many other people's babies, finally I had my son in my arms. It was terrifying and amazing, and nothing was ever the same from that moment onwards. Not one thing. Motherhood has changed every fibre of my being."

For her second child, Jessie, Catherine chose to give birth in

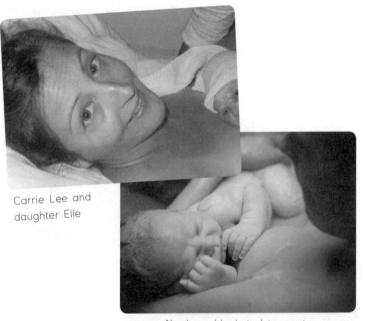

Carrie Lee and
daughter Elle

Newborn blanketed in vernix

a unit run by midwives. "It was the most beautiful experience possible. I knew what I was doing, and so did Jessie. She came out softly and gently, in her own sweet time. Her gorgeous, warm loveliness filled the room and we all fell in love. I fed her for forty minutes just after she was born, and she fitted perfectly into this Jessie-sized space in our lives that we hadn't known was there."

Says Catherine, "I still love thinking about those moments, when these wonderful people arrived and everything changed."

Much of a mother's feeling of "falling in love" at first sight with her baby is linked to the combination of hormones cascading through her body. The love hormone oxytocin increases during labour and peaks around the time of childbirth. But it isn't alone: prolactin, known as the "hormone of surrender", peaks then too. When prolactin surges in a chimpanzee, it makes a male cower before the troop leader, and it seems that the hormone helps ensure both parents submit to their baby's every cry and call.

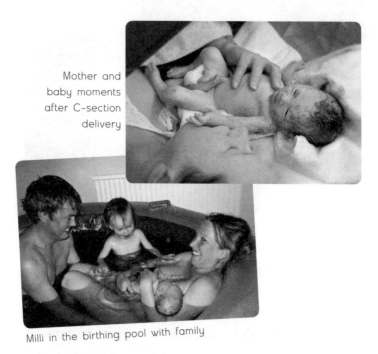

Mother and baby moments after C-section delivery

Milli in the birthing pool with family

For me, giving birth was touching the face of God, or of eternity.

– *Suzanne Stalls, New Mexico, USA*

A magic moment

"When my husband, Nick, and I found out I was pregnant with our first boy, George, we were so thrilled," says Emily Eavis, co-organizer of the Glastonbury Festival and White Ribbon Alliance Champion in the UK. "I'd had a miscarriage previously, which I found quite hard to deal with, so getting pregnant again meant a lot but also came with a fair share of worry.

"As we ticked off the weeks, we got more confident that we were going to be okay and I loved being pregnant. We moved house twice during that time, and in both my pregnancies I remember feeling this enormous strength, like I could carry several huge boxes at once. People would say, 'Oh no, be careful, don't lift anything!' But it gives you such an enormous rush of power and strength!

"Seeing our babies' faces for the first time brought both me and Nick to tears. It's totally indescribable the feeling you have, the deep well of love you have for your children.

"Now we have two children – the younger, Noah, is six months – and both have arrived in time for the Glastonbury Festival; I'm sure it's all a plan, because they just don't want to miss out. Balancing the organization of the festival with children requires a fair amount of juggling, but my husband and I share of lot of the childcare and I think it would be impossible to do it without that."

Emily's babies were born within weeks and months of the children of several close friends, some of whom she went to school with and who now also work at the festival. For Emily, it has made a huge difference: "Being able to share all of this with close friends means so much; we are all like a big family, supporting each other on a daily basis. I'll always remember us sitting around with our feet up high, exhausted, legs swollen and cabbage leaves [soothing when breast-feeding] in our bras, laughing in our shared discomfort! Being in close proximity to friends or family is paramount, I think, and having children growing up together is really special – they already have such great friendships, which I think is the cornerstone to everything in life.

"Having babies gives you an underlying sense of what really is important. What would once have sent us over the edge no longer does. It just doesn't have the same importance."

✻ ✻ ✻ ✻

A lass if born in June with a caul
Will wed, hev bairns & rear 'em all.
But a lass if born with a caul in July,
Will loose her caul & young will die.
Every month beside luck comes with a caul
If safe put by,
If lost she may cry:
For ill luck on her will fall.
For man it's luck – be born when he may –
It is safe be kept ye mind,
But if lost it be he'll find
Ill-deed his lot for many a day

– Traditional rhyme collected in 1875,
Pitt Rivers Museum, University of Oxford

Born with a caul

"I was born with a caul, which was advertised for sale, in the newspapers, at the low price of fifteen guineas," declares David Copperfield, eponymous hero of Charles Dickens' novel. "Whether sea going people were short of money about that time, or were short of faith and preferred cork jackets, I don't know...", but, sadly for young David, there were no takers at this price.

It was thought in Dickens' time that a child born with a caul – a part of the amniotic sac still attached to the head or face, which happens in about one out of a thousand births – would never die of drowning. Cauls could fetch a good price at auction, bought by sailors as a lucky charm. A child born with a caul was also thought to have "second sight", special powers of perception.

Dickens clearly took this popular superstition with a pinch of salt: eventually, the caul was raffled, and won "by an old lady with a hand-basket who very reluctantly produced from it the stipulated five shillings," continues David. "It is a fact that will long be remembered that she was never drowned but died triumphantly in her bed at ninety-two. I have understood that it was to the last her proudest boast that she never had been on the water in her life, except upon a bridge..."

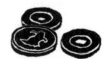

18

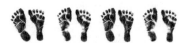

SWEET WHISPERS:
AL-TAHNEEK (ISLAM)

Straight after my baby Kamran was born, his dad whispered the *adhan* (أذان) in his ear," remembers Sarah Javaid, who lives in London, where she co-founded MADE (Muslim Agency for Development Education) in Europe with her husband, Nadeem. *Allah Akbar. La ilaha illa Allah. Sashadu anna Muhammadan Rasool Allah. Hayya 'alas-Salah.* "God is great. There is no God but Allah. Muhammad is the messenger of Allah. Come to prayer."

Sarah explains: "The *adhan* is the call to prayer, which Muslims around the world hear five times a day, an affirmation of our faith in one God and the Prophet Muhammad (PBUH). Our custom is for this to be the first thing that a newborn baby hears when she enters the world."

For Muslim families like Sarah's, the tradition offers clear guidance on the first words a baby will hear. Without that custom to steer him, Reg Matheson spontaneously welcomed his daughter using the name he and his wife had decided before her birth, saying, "You're here, Dusty Rose, you're here." But you may not know your child's gender, or you may not yet have considered, let alone decided upon, a name. Indeed, many parents say they are completely at a loss for words when their newborn emerges into the world.

The moment of birth is such a precious time, a rare experience in any parent's life. What first words will you speak to your baby?

My child, you have been born from our heart. May you live a hundred years and see a hundred autumns, may you have a long and glorious life, overcoming all ills and enjoying complete happiness, prosperity and fortune.

— *Tibetan prayer traditionally spoken to the newborn*

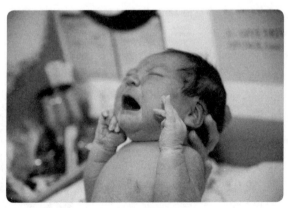

Hello baby

The healing date

In Islam, the date – also known as the "bread of the desert" – is considered an especially important food; dates are said to be the food of Paradise.

The Qur'an tells how God instructed Maryam, as she neared the time for the birth of 'Isa (Jesus) and was overwhelmed by the pain, to "shake towards you the trunk of the palm tree and it will drop on you fresh ripe dates. So eat, drink and be consoled." When a woman is pregnant, it was believed that the easily absorbed sugar in dates would help facilitate contractions and birth.

In *Kitab Al-Taharah*, or *The Book of Purification*, Hadith 560 reveals how, after blessing them, the Prophet Muhammad rubbed the mouth of infants with a well-chewed date – a practice called *al-tahneek* (ل-تهنيق). It was said that *tahneek* could imbue the child with the qualities of a virtuous person. Today, it is also said that rubbing a paste made from a fresh date on a baby's gums or palate will help kick-start the digestive system.

As it happens, doctors at Leeds General Infirmary in England have reported that giving babies a small dose of sugar syrup (about two millilitres) before their first blood test reduces crying time.

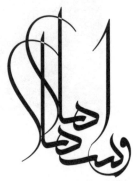

The Arabic "welcome"

19

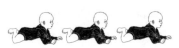

WHENUA: HOME FOR THE "SECOND" BABY (MAORI)

The labour is finally done, and at last the baby has been born. Everyone, especially the mother, is exhausted and delighted – but it's not over. Some minutes later, there is a second, necessary delivery: the placenta.

First-time mothers are sometimes taken by surprise when the placenta arrives. They have their baby in their arms, and yet more contractions are coming – although these feel more like cramps and are far less intense than the contractions of labour. The placenta is also quite large, which may be why many cultures call it the "second baby". Fortunately, it is also soft and pliable, and the bliss of seeing the baby means most women don't mind a bit of extra work at this point. However, it is essential that every bit of the placenta is delivered, as any bits left attached to the wall of the uterus can cause heavy bleeding.

There is now a decision to be made: what to do with this tissue that has nurtured the baby for so long? For many women around the world, the placenta's role in keeping the baby alive and well means that it must be treated with respect, whether the birth has taken place in a hospital or on the floor of your home.

Back to the land

In the Māori language, the word for "land" and the word for "placenta" are the same: *whenua*. According to traditional Māori folklore, all life is born from *papatūānuku*, the womb of the Earth, which is located under the sea. The land is a life-giving force – as is the placenta – so, when a baby is born, the mother must bury the placenta in the earth.

This practice was thought to reinforce the vital relationship between the people and their land – linking them to their original home, ensuring they would not abandon the place where they were born.

Mandy Briggs recalls: "My daughter was born in New Zealand at a friend's farmhouse, and when I took her home I took the placenta with me in a container and kept it in the fridge. When I had recovered from the birth, we walked up to the ridge behind my house, found a spot with a wonderful view and buried it in the ground. I planted a little sapling on top.

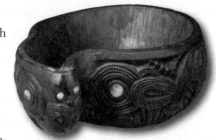

"My friend gave birth soon after, and she did the same on the hillside opposite to where I had buried mine. She also planted a tree, and whenever I go back I visit her

A Māori *ipu whenua*, or placenta bowl

and we go up and see our children's trees. I'm happy to think that – even when we are far from 'home' – their trees are looking at each other across the valley, and will be for many years to come."

The second baby

In southern Africa, the Xhosa believe that the burying of the placenta, called *inkaba*, attaches the baby to her ancestral lands and clan. Later in life, a person returns to this burial spot to communicate hopes and dreams to her ancestors.

"The placenta is tightly guarded; it is precious," says Samuel Senfuka, a chief of the Buganda people of Uganda. "Traditionally, it was buried under a special banana tree near the woman's home."

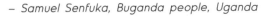

> It is believed that the tree where the placenta is buried holds special blessings for the baby as it grows.
> – *Samuel Senfuka, Buganda people, Uganda*

Samuel goes on: "Alternatively, women would sometimes bury the placenta near the doorway of their house. This is in order to remove it from the reach of people with evil purposes. People in communities and even in the family often have their differences, and women may fear that someone would want to use the placenta to kill their child, or render the mother unable to conceive again, through witchcraft. They believe that, if their enemies get hold of the placenta, they could use its powers for these bad purposes."

Samuel says this often influences choices about how women give birth in his country. "This is one of the reasons why some women still avoid delivering in hospitals and clinics, because the placenta is thrown in a 'placenta pit' to avoid infection. Because women do not get to take possession of their placenta in hospitals, they choose to give birth in their own homes, without medical help – which can be very dangerous. People often think women are not going to health centres because there is a shortage of midwives, poor conditions or lack of supplies, but loss of the placenta is an important factor."

The power of the placenta

According to Rebecca Tortello, author of *Pieces of the Past*, people take special measures to protect the placenta, burying it in special or sacred locations in accordance with ancient rituals.

✷ The origin of the soul (Cambodia): In rural parts of the country, the placenta is known as "the globe of the origin of the soul", and people believe it should be buried in a special location, the spot protected with a spiky plant to keep evil spirits (and dogs!) from interfering with its rest. If this is done well, it is a good omen for the mother's mental health.

✷ The source of piety (Turkey): If Turkish parents wish their child to be devout, they may bury the placenta in the courtyard of a mosque.

✷ Count on future siblings (Ukraine): Tradition holds that a midwife could divine from the placenta how many more children the mother would bear. The placenta was later buried in a place where it would not be stepped over. If it was buried under the doorway, it was said the mother would become infertile.

⬧ Opt for a last birth (Transylvania): If a couple desired not to have any more children, they would burn their baby's placenta and mix it with ashes. Then, to render himself infertile, the husband would drink this potent mixture.

⬧ Poke away evil (Persia): In a practice that may have Zoroastrian roots, the placenta was poked with a needle to frighten evil spirits called *al* that are associated with harm to the mother or newborn. Then the placenta was buried with a piece of charcoal to discourage animals from digging it up.

⬧ Feed the spirit (Bali): The Balinese believe that every child has four invisible siblings – conceived and born at the same time as the baby. They are represented by the amniotic fluid, the uterine blood, the *vernix caseoasa* (the waxy substance that covers the baby at birth) and the placenta. At birth, the father collects the *ari-ari*, or placenta, washes it, places it in a coconut with flowers and money, and wraps the coconut in a white cloth before burying it outside the family's home. The burial is marked with a large black rock and a pandanus bush, and is meant to protect the child throughout his life. When the mother feeds the baby, it is said that some drops of milk should be spilled on the burial site to feed the four siblings – if they are not treated well, they may lash out at the child.

The child's spirit helpers

Among some of the First Nations people of what is now Canada, when the woman's water broke everyone would come and touch the water and bless themselves with it, like it was holy water because it came from such a pure place where the unborn child was growing.

The placenta was cared for also; it wasn't just thrown away. Different peoples had different traditions about that: some would bury it; some would burn it; some would wrap it and place it high up in a tree somewhere far out in the bush so that the animals and birds would take it and in turn they would become the child's spirit helpers. Sometimes it was the father's responsibility to take care of it; this was an important part of ensuring the health and spiritual well-being of the child.

— Lesley Paulette, Aboriginal midwife, Northwest Territories, Canada

20

JUBILATIONS AND THANKSGIVINGS:
A MOMENT TO PAUSE

After hours of intensely hard labour, the baby has at last been born. The expression on the face of the new mother is indescribable; the word "joy" only comes close.

Finally, the waiting is over, and hopefully mother and baby are doing well. In many cultures, there now follows a period of seclusion, rest and recuperation for the mother – but, at the same time, the rest of the community cannot wait to express their delight. But who will spread the news and how?

Different cultures have their own long-established ways of announcing the birth and welcoming both child and new mother, but it is always a big moment. In some countries, it is often only a matter of hours (or minutes!) before a photo drops into the email inbox of friends and relatives, showing the ecstatic parents' faces hovering over an oblivious newborn, who does not yet know the sparkling, inescapable attraction of a smartphone.

In other countries, news travels by word of mouth – and much of the news involves letting people know that now there is much

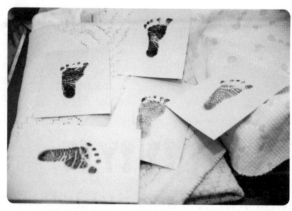

Inked foot prints in delivery room

to be done to care for the mother and baby, beginning with the first blessings for a long, good life.

Let good things happen to me

"In my village, when a baby is born, the good news is spread to the immediate family, who in turn invite their extended family members and neighbours by chanting songs, which indicate that a new child is born," says Lizzy Agams of the Igbo people of Nigeria.

"Celebration of childbirth is the first of a series of rites of passage; people gather and sing for joy, thanking God for the new arrival, congratulating the mother for doing a good job, the father for doing even a greater one. So many songs are rendered during the celebration of a newborn." Often, she says, the community will sing *Oma merem merem merem* ("Let good things happen to me") or *Nwayi tupu muru, ina tupu ina a muru* ("Woman conceive and give birth").

Sixth-day festivities

Deepa Jha of White Ribbon Alliance India lives in Delhi. She recalls how her family gathered around her for her baby's birth. "Before the birth and for three months afterwards, I went to stay with my parents in Jharkhand; I wanted to have family and friends around me. I was able to have complete rest, and my family took such good care of me and the baby.

"Five days after my son was born, we held the *chatti* ceremony [*chhah* (छह) means "six" in Hindi, for the sixth day of the baby's life]. It was a party for all the family, held at the house of my husband's parents. I had a brand-new sari, and my son had a special outfit, all in yellow, which is an auspicious colour.

"During the ceremony, I took my baby on my lap and I performed the *puja*, saying prayers to the gods for him to have a long and healthy life. Our guests blessed me and our new child."

The *chatti* is also a time for naming the child, Deepa explains. "According to tradition, it is the husband's elder sister who proposes the name of the new baby. She had checked with us beforehand and we were happy with her proposal, so at the ceremony it was announced that our son would be called Akchat.

"And then we had a feast, with lots of good home-cooked food!"

✳ ✳ ✳ ✳ ✳ ✳ ✳ ✳ ✳ ✳ ✳ ✳ ✳ ✳

"Baby Blessing", from Petals of Poetry

It was the laughter of a child
On mama's lap
That brought tears to my heart
Innocence so profound
Wealth unimaginable
Purity plus

It was such vulnerability
Fortified in absolute dependence
Of one so genuine
So resolute in the belief
Mama holds me
That churned my soul

It was the gentle stubbornness
Of strength in weakness
The catch me if you can run
Wind-power willpower
That got me wondering
What it would be like

It was the thrill in the voice
As mama bit the little ears
Her face pride beaming
Filled with satisfaction
For the prized possession
That meant the world

It was the dance of God
That I saw in His heart
As He scooped the little legs
Thrown in the air, assurance
That Daddy wouldn't let me fall
That made me desire my own

Desire my own despite a painful past
Of mama losing child after child
For far flung hospitals
Prime poverty plots
A commitment that because I lived
Mine would live.

– *Larry Liza, White Ribbon Alliance champion,
Nairobi, Kenya*

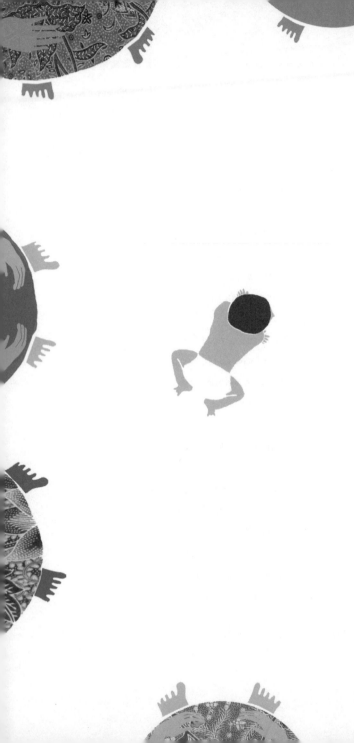

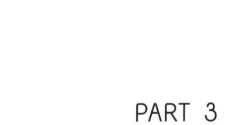

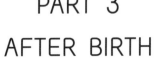

PART 3
AFTER BIRTH

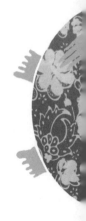

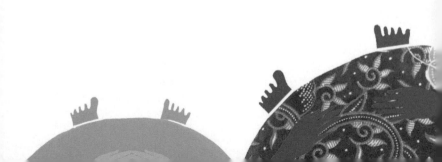

PART 3

AFTER BIRTH

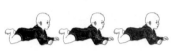

21

A NEW *EKYOGERO*
FOR GRANDMOTHER (UGANDA)

Contrary to popular belief (most especially among young people), getting older can be really great. In fact, plenty of studies have shown that the older you get – as long as you have good health – the happier you are. And, having put the years of childbearing behind them, many older women have a great longing to become grandmothers.

How wonderful to share in the joys of holding a newborn without the tiredness of the new mother. How delightful to feed and bathe, care for and play with that growing child, building on experience gained long ago and now revitalized in creating a precious new relationship.

At the same time, it has dawned on the new mother for the first time just what her own mother went through in carrying her, giving birth and raising her to adulthood. There is often a renewed bond between mother and daughter, inspired by respect and shared affection.

Grandmothers are also an invaluable source of wisdom and experience, especially when medical care is hard to reach.

A helping pair of hands

"In our Buganda culture, the husband will immediately spread news of the birth to all the relatives. The grandmother will be the first to bathe the newborn and to give her blessings to the new mother," says Samuel Senfuka of Uganda. "The grandmother will immediately prepare herbs for bathing the baby.

"The family will buy a new saucepan, never used before, known as an *ekyogero*, and put herbs in it with water. Some of the herbs include *ebbombo* (to cure cough), *kayayana* (to be loved by everyone) and *omwolola* and *olumanyo* (for knowledge)." Other herbs added to the bath may be *olweza* (to bring good luck), *bbombo* (to cure fevers) and *namirembe* (for calming). "Every morning and evening, the grandmother will warm the mixture and bathe the baby in the herbs; she will also give the baby some droplets of the same herbs."

Some Buganda people say the grandmother should give the first bath because she is more careful than others.

Blessed and valued

But the baby is not the only one to receive care. "The woman is taken care of by her husband's female relatives, such as the mother-in-law or sister-in-law. They will take care of her for the first two weeks after the birth. She receives a lot of care and love at this time," Samuel says. "They prepare special meals for her such as porridge, offal and eggplants for boosting breast milk.

She also is bathed in herbs. This helps her body – her private parts and her stomach – to recover and regain their shape. She is cared for because they value her life.

"She will have many visitors – relatives, aunties, friends – all coming to congratulate her and to thank her for giving a child to the clan. They bring gifts for the woman and the newborn – clothes, money, food and handcrafts. There are many jubilations and celebrations!

"People believe the herbal mixture gives blessings to the mother and baby, prevents illness and infections, protects against skin rashes and helps give shape and form to the newborn," Samuel explains. Later, if the child's head is too big or too soft, or if the waist is not in proportion, the people of the village will say it is because the baby didn't get enough of the herbs – that is, care from his grandmother."

Three generations

Birth can send the whole family into a spin; usual routines are disrupted, sleep times and meals can suffer, emotions are running high. This is when a helpful grandmother, skilled, tactful and practised in holding a family together, can be invaluable.

"After the birth, the mother of the bride purchases foodstuffs, herbs and spices, and she goes to spend a minimum of one month and a maximum of three months with her daughter to take care of her and the newborn. This visit is called *omugwo*," explains Lizzy Agams of the Igbo people of Nigeria.

"When the mother arrives, she assumes the duties of mother and babysitter; she cooks for the household, massages the new mother with hot water and local ointments so that her body can come back to normal." Many will prepare *ji mmili oku uda* [yam pepper soup] with West African peppers called *uda* and *uziza*, which are said to help with healing. "The grandmother also bathes the newborn baby because her daughter, the new mother, cannot handle the delicate baby at that point in time," Lizzy says.

"The first day this new baby comes into our homes, he or she will be carried around the house as a sign of welcome. The baby will be seated on the bare floor as a sign of acceptance by all – and to say to the ancestors, 'We have increased by one or two', as the case may be. Pregnancy and childbirth are cherished and highly celebrated, because this is a thing of joy."

Omugwo is so beloved that Nigerian families around the world continue the tradition.

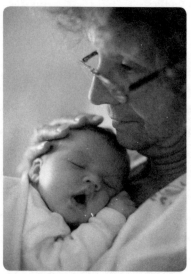

Sleeping baby in grandmother's arms, France

A grandfather's revelation

Becoming a grandparent is wonderful. It's quite intriguing; maybe it's biological. You feel this deep fondness, you want to smother them with affection and help them with everything. People say it's because you can "take them back", but that's got nothing to do with it.

With your own children, you're often in the wrong, or you're not like someone else's dad...whereas your grandchildren just adore you for who you are. They have a blind faith in you but your own children are more realistic. It is very entertaining most of the time; sometimes they can be a bit of a pain. There are funny moments when you mutter to yourself, "Oh, sod it" or "Oh God", and the grandchildren reply, "What was that, Grandpa...?" You have to be careful what you say, because they copy everything you do.

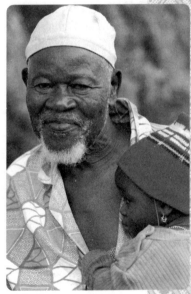

It's a very strange thing and I feel rather guilty – *Why wasn't I like this for my own children?* But really, being a grandparent is unbelievable. I didn't expect to feel like this at all.

– Michael Eavis, dairy farmer and co-organizer of the Glastonbury Festival, UK

Elder with baby, Burkina Faso

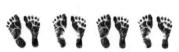

22

OUTCOMING:
MEETING THE FAMILY (CAMBODIA)

Kiev Martin says that spirits are still very present in her Cambodian family's thinking when it comes to rituals and celebrations: "We still believe that the spirits guide us and watch over us. For instance, when my family lived on the Cambodian border, the Khmer Rouge came to rob us. My grandmother had passed away by then, and her ashes were hung from the middle beam of our family hut. We were storing two sewing machines in our hut for the community, but if the Khmer had found them we would have been considered very rich and could have been killed. Although the soldiers searched and found others things we had hidden, like sarongs and watches, they never saw the sewing machines at the end of our bamboo bed covered with my mother's sarong. My family believes this was because the spirit of my grandmother blinded them from seeing the sewing machines, even in a hut that was only five by five meters.

"My own mother is still very traditional. She never got the chance to go to school after sixth grade. By the age of twelve, she had to run her own business to contribute to her family. They left Cambodia as refugees and arrived in America with nothing but a trash bag of old clothes. She couldn't speak English, but she worked making take-away food. She is a strong woman with a lot of common sense."

Calling on the ancestors

So, when the one-month anniversary of Kiev's sons' births arrived, she knew a traditional and very spiritual "outcoming" ceremony was expected. This is when the extended family and community of friends are first "invited to meet the baby". The baby is now healthy enough to be showered with presents. "Everybody gives the baby money and jewellery – such as gold anklets, bracelets or necklaces," says Kiev. At her sons' outcomings, they had about one hundred guests – "which is considered a small group in our tradition".

There are also many contemplative moments. "We light the 'big candle', which is made of one hundred percent beeswax – it

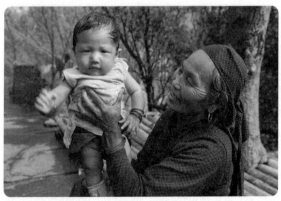

Grandmother celebrating her grandchild, Nepal

was the same candle used in my wedding. The candle is placed on a table as a way of inviting your ancestors to the ceremony and signifies the spirit. It is laid out in a special way, with welcoming drinks such as tea and whisky, and twelve types of food, with chopsticks, for the ancestors to enjoy. Those foods include long noodles, symbolizing long life, and ball-shaped desserts, symbolizing the unity within the family."

Our ancestors, especially the great-grandparents who have passed away, join the event, sit and have a drink – and take away a "goody bag" of food when they go.
– *Kiev Martin, Maryland, USA*

For the outcoming, the baby has a first haircut and is cared for in other ways. "My son's head was shaved by my father, so that his hair would grow quicker and thicker. My mother applied Tiger Balm [a menthol rub] to his stomach in order to prevent stomach upsets. (She would have done this every day until he was two years old, but she had to go back to Cambodia!)"

This is also the time when a child's name is revealed to everyone. "The names are selected by the grandfather," Kiev explains. Her sons received Chinese names – Shunheng and Shunlong – and also English names, Steven and Thomas, given to them by their dad who is American.

"My elder son's Chinese name is Shunheng meaning peaceful and luck. He is a peacemaker wherever he goes. So I am very lucky. My younger son's Chinese name means peaceful and loud;

needless to say, wherever he goes, you will remember him."

She adds: "I was raised as a Buddhist and we continue the Cambodian traditions, but I have been baptized as a Presbyterian in America, and I will have my sons baptized if we can get all our family in one place."

A full member of the clan

"After the baby is born, the mother will keep and carefully preserve the umbilical cord. Then, a year or more later, or whenever there is a last funeral rite among the husband's family, the child is taken to be initiated into the clan, known as *omwâná*," says Samuel Senfuka, a chief of the Buganda people of Uganda.

"In a ritual that takes place in front of clan members, the grandparents and aunties will put water in a bucket, then take the umbilical cord, smeared with butter, and immerse it in the water. If it floats, this confirms that the child does belong to the clan and not to another man's family."

Family offerings

In Moldova, after the child is born, the father-in-law traditionally was expected to bring the new mother a chicken with black feathers tied with a red bow, as well as vodka. The mother-in-law would give earrings for a baby girl or a ring for a baby boy. The child's godmother would cut the baby's nails and hair for the first time, and leave some money by the child's pillow.

Samuel admits that the tradition can be nerve-wracking. "At this time, the mother does feel very tense and nervous in case the cord sinks! If it sinks, she will always be asked to be honest and mention the true father of the child. If it happens that it belongs to another man, arrangements are done to take the child to the true father after he compensates for all the costs incurred by the woman's husband. And, when the cord is seen to float in the water, the people will clap, beat drums, eat, dance – and congratulate the mother. More jubilations!" A few days later the child is named – the *okwálúlá omwâná*.

In any case, says Samuel, "These traditions are a way of preventing harm to the community and to the woman. They make people feel safe and that they belong to the family. They are a way of raising children with good behaviour."

Birthday bake off

An Albanian tradition says that, on day three of the baby's life, you bake pastries and give them to friends and family. This shows your gratefulness for the life of the newborn.
– Sharlene Daly, midwife, UK

Stepping into the world

I am Yoruba and one of our most important traditions is the baby's first bath. There is great importance attached to this first bath; we believe that, if not done properly, issues with hygiene will follow the baby throughout life. The task is usually entrusted to an elderly woman in the family, or a trusted elder woman, and it is believed that this process signifies the child stepping into the world.

For the bath, *ose dudu*, a traditional herbal soap made from shea butter, camwood, honey, lemon and other herbs, is prepared. It clarifies and cleanses the newborn baby's skin, removing the vernix. During the bath, the baby is moved suddenly and rapidly, as we believe this experience prepares the child for the unexpected hardships of life.

A naming ceremony is held on the eighth day after birth for girls, and on the seventh day after birth for boys. As part of the ceremony, the baby is given a mixture of sugar, signifying sweet life; salt, signifying an enjoyable life; palm oil, signifying an easy life, free of difficulties; and water, the source of life. The names given to a child usually reflect the circumstances leading to the birth of the baby – her pedigree, antecedents and, most importantly, her parents' aspirations.

Names are submitted to the religious clerics officiating over the naming ceremony by members of the family and well-wishers. My name, Oluwatosin, is a Christian name inspired by Psalm 116:9, "I will walk before the Lord in the land of the living" and Colossians 1:10, "That ye might walk worthy of the Lord unto all pleasing, be-ing fruitful in every good work, and increasing in the knowledge of God." My Muslim name, Halimat, was in-spired by Halimah Saa'diyah, the foster mother and wet nurse for the Prophet Muhammad (PBUH).

The birth of a child in my country is always welcomed with joy, yet there are still high mortality rates. I feel very lucky to be part of the movement to reduce death in childbirth and help babies survive.

– *Tosin Saraki, Wellbeing Foundation, Nigeria*

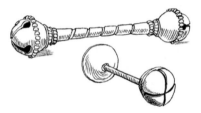

A welcoming ceremony

Interfaith minister Vera Waters has created a special ceremony to "bring out" a new baby to any community. To begin, she invites family and friends into a circle, then calls on the Divine to be present and shares these words:

Gods of our home, gods of the home of this baby, gods of the hearth, today we present you with someone new.

She is a member of our family, and she is welcome to join us to celebrate the gift of life.

We ask you to welcome her, we ask you to love her, we ask you to protect her, and we ask you to bless her.

Next, a cup of water is passed around, and each member of the family takes a sip. When the cup returns to Vera, she takes a drop of water from the cup and touches it to the baby's lips. The participants are asked to hold hands as Vera says:

Gods of this home, gods of our hearth, today we present you with someone new.

She is a member of our family, and she is a gift from God.

Watch over her as she grows.

Watch over her as she lives.

Watch over her with Love.

Then she asks the baby's loved ones to join her in prayer:

Great Spirit, Source of All, we ask for your blessing on the arrival of this baby into this family and home.

We give thanks for the great miracle of birth and remember your gift of breath, the gift of life.

May this family be united in love for the joy of knowing that this baby has come to join them and to bring her own special skills, wisdom and knowledge to them.

May their joy continue as she grows up and becomes the great light that shines upon them all.

Dear Great One, blessings and thanks for uniting the family and we remember our ancestors, those who have walked before us on this earthly plane.

We especially remember the women of this family who have lived before and who guide and support the new life of this baby.

One of the parents steps forward to read a poem. A particular favourite is "On Children", from *The Prophet* by Kahlil Gibran:

Your children are not your children
They are the sons and daughters of Life's longing for itself.
They come through you but not from you.
And though they are with you yet they belong not to you.
You may give them your Love but not your thoughts.
For they have their own thoughts.
You may house their bodies but not their souls.
For their souls dwell in the house of tomorrow,

which you cannot visit, even in your Dreams.

You may strive to be like them,

But seek not to make them like you.

For life goes not backward nor tarries with yesterday.

You are the bows from which your children

As living arrows are sent forth.

Then the other parent is invited to say a few words or recite a poem.

Vera describes what comes next: "I invite the rest of the family to speak from their hearts, and for the children to bring their drawings. I pass the cup around one more time, with each person offering a blessing as they sip the water. Once the cup has returned to me, I touch another drop of water to the baby's lips. The cup is left on the table (decorated with flowers and candles, like an altar) overnight as an offering to the baby's spirit guardians. The parents are invited to take the cup outside in the morning and pour what is left onto the ground, as an offering to the spirits of nature."

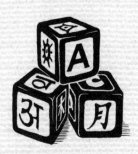

23

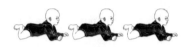

SMOKING THE BABY (ABORIGINAL PEOPLE, AUSTRALIA)

Midwife Rachael Lockey moved to Alice Springs, Australia, in 2007. She went there to work at a women's health and maternity centre, a branch of the Central Australian Aboriginal Congress, located on the outskirts of town, on land that was traditionally a women's place.

"I was very excited when the plane touched down," she recalls. "I'd come from a busy, densely populated island called Great Britain. And as I came off the plane, across the tarmac, I was struck by the scent of native plants, the plants of central Australia, the desert. Astringent, sharp tones, fresh and uplifting with some softness added by their blooms.

"It was soon revealed to me that Alice is not in fact in the middle of nowhere but in the middle of everywhere!" she says. Some of the communities served by the town's centre were nearly eight hundred miles away. These were often small villages or towns, numbering anywhere from fifty to a thousand people. Places with "beautiful names like Titjikala, Papunya, Alpurrurulam,

Areyonga, each with its own people, own tribe, own language and own ways".

Rachael remembers settling into her new work. "In many ways, midwifery in such a different setting was reassuringly familiar to me. The usual schedule of pregnancy visits, hospital for birthing, some home births, postnatal visits. And yet I had arrived in a different world."

Infused with old wisdom

The smoking ceremony is a cultural tradition among the Aboriginal people across Australia. The ceremony is typically held both at birth and at death. Rachael learned that it was part of the routine for all of the clinic's patients.

"The leadership at the *alukura* [an Arrente word meaning 'place for woman and children'] made it a must!" she says. "No regular clinic on smoking-ceremony days – just all staff on deck, along with the grandmothers and aunties, the holders of women's law and culture.

"Branches of shrubs, bushes and trees, specially selected for their healing properties, were placed together in a shallow pit and lit to start a fire. The flame dies down quickly to a smoulder, then the smoke rises slowly and purposefully."

> The scent of the place, of the land, of leaves, is released, filling the air.
>
> – *Rachael Lockey, midwife*

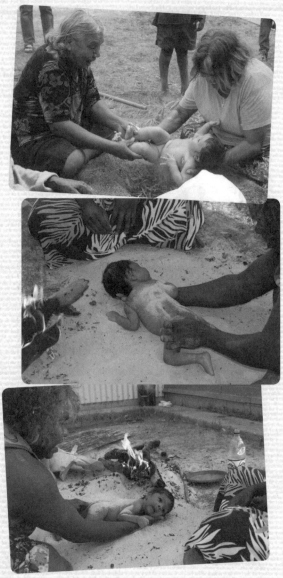

Arrente baby smoking ceremony

"A brand-new little one, a few weeks or a few months old, is passed over the smoke in the trusted hands of the grandmothers [the elder women of the community]. The baby is turned over and around and upside down. The mother leans over the smoke, with grandmothers on either side of her and her breasts exposed. There is believed to be a connection between breastfeeding, milk supply and the ritual of smoking."

Gathering the sacred smoke

After the smoking of the mother and baby, everyone in attendance is invited to lean into the smoke, Rachael says. This is so they can "experience the smoke rising up across your body, over your face and through your hair, and to benefit from the purifying and protective elements held within the plants," she says. "Finally, the billy [a tin case used for heating water over a fire] boils and the campfire tea is made."

Rachael goes on: "In many urban environments, where we are constantly confronted with modernity, technology, information overload, business and medicalization, the practice of cultural traditions has become less common. What I learned from these times was how open women are to sharing precious occasions such as these. There is a universal culture of childbirth, the great significance of bringing another into the world, that unites us."

✖ ✖ ✖ ✖

Extra care

In communities without antibiotics for newborn infections, there are many herbal and other traditional healing practices used to care for babies.

✦ Smoke the fear out (Xhosa, southern Africa): The traditional midwife prepares a mixture of ash, sugar and mashed fruit of the *umtuma*, a noxious plant. After the baby's birth, a piece of sharp dry grass is used to cut the cord, and some hours later the potion is applied to the remaining umbilicus, so that it will dry and fall off within a few days. Now, the mother and child are allowed to spend time with the women of her community. Soon afterwards, the child will go through the ritual of *sifudu*, which involves holding the baby in the smoke of pungent *sifudu* tree leaves before passing her under the mother's knees, one after the other. This is meant to keep the child from being timid or easily frightened – to be strong in spirit.

✦ Cure with spice (Cambodia): It is traditional to make a poultice from ginger to place on the umbilicus and stomach to encourage healing.

✦ Cure with herbs (Somalia): Newborns are given warm baths and massages with sesame oil during which the infant's limbs are stretched gently. A herb, *malmal*, is applied to the umbilicus for the first week of life – it is said to protect the baby from the "evil eye". The mother would often wear a bracelet of *malmal* too. The baby's clothing and bedding are also placed on a wooden rack and stretched over burning frankincense, so that the cleansing, aromatic fumes infuse the cloth – and fill the home.

Keeping the sweepings

Following birth, a Jamaican "nana", or midwife, traditionally dressed the child's navel with nutmeg. She would blow smoke into the child's eyes, often from an old clay pipe. The nana would then wash her own face with rum. Sometimes she would down a stiff drink to improve her "eyesight", since the witnessing of each birth was said to affect her sight.

The mother and child were often isolated for nine days, during which time the nana took control of the house. It was considered very important to protect mother and child from spiritual harm and any physical dangers.

The mother had to wear sanitary pads made from new pieces of cloth and the house was kept closed – all air holes were blocked with either pieces of cloth or paper to keep out breezes. She would tie red cloth on the infant to keep away evil spirits.

A special broom was used to sweep out the room and the sweepings were kept, perhaps to prevent others from getting hold of them for witchcraft. The child was marked with blue, and the pair of scissors or knife used to cut the umbilical cord was watched carefully. Some sort of *guzu*, or charm – often a strong-smelling substance – was also used to protect the child.

The baby was washed in cold water containing rum and a silver coin given by the father. The water and coin were later buried in the yard, along with the afterbirth. The nana counted the knots on the umbilical cord to determine how many children the mother was destined to have.

On the tenth day, the mother and child were taken outside to receive greetings as well as presents from family members and other visitors. The child was named on that day. This practice is believed to have come from the West African belief that, until day eight, the child's fate is uncertain and his personality/soul is not fully formed. In addition, there was the possibility that the child could be a visitor from the spiritual world, and, if that was the case, then he must not be welcomed. If the child died during this period, for example, it was believed that an evil spirit had arrived.

These rituals are said to be similar to those practised by the earliest Jamaicans, the Tainos. Although no records of Jamaican rituals exist from this period, in Guyana, where there are some direct descendants of Tainos, a child is not regarded as an individual separate from his mother for the first five to twelve days of life. Both mother and baby are considered polluted and kept indoors to prevent contamination. The naming ceremony takes place ten to twelve days following birth.

– *Dr Rebecca Tortello, author of* Pieces of the Past

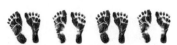

24

LATCHING ON:
A TIME OF RICHES (NEPAL)

It is a kind of miracle: a woman brings new life into the world, and immediately she has the power to nourish, comfort and satisfy her baby at her breast. No wonder many peoples celebrate the life-giving properties of breast milk!

The ancient Greeks believed that the stars of the Milky Way were formed from the droplets of Hera's breast milk. Artemis of Ephesus – who had many breasts – was revered as the source of abundance and fertility for all life on Earth. The Egyptian goddess Hathor, worshipped as creator of the universe, was depicted as a cow with kings suckling at her udders.

In Christianity, the milk of Mary, mother of Jesus, has been described as an emanation from heaven, a balm for the soul, a symbol of love, wisdom, mercy and healing. Many cultures through the ages have stories on the same theme, from the Roman legend of imprisoned Micon, who was saved from starvation by his daughter Pero's breast milk, to Rose of Sharon in John Steinbeck's *The Grapes of Wrath*, who saves a dying man by feeding him from her breast after her own baby dies.

Breast milk has anti-viral properties and has long been used as a medicine for ailments ranging from deafness to snakebite. Women in many countries use drops of breast milk to treat "sticky eye" infections in their newborn. And, in Nepal, some women don't just feed the baby with breast milk; they also massage it into their skin to promote good health.

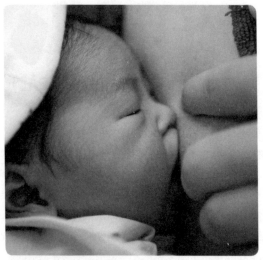

Getting the position right

Strengthening the mother

"In Nepal, there is a praiseworthy culture of supporting the new mother as she breastfeeds her child. This is seen as a matter of top priority and great importance," says Samjhana Phuyal.

"After the birth, the mother is given very nutritious foods to make sure she can produce enough breast milk; she will be given chicken soup, mutton broth or *jwanu ko jhwoli* [lovage soup]. She is given a special kind of herbal medicine, made from a range of spices, often in the form of sweets."

To help the mother and baby relax, they are both given a hot oil massage – the paternal grandmother of the baby taking responsibility for the care of the baby. Then, eleven days after the birth, mother and baby go to stay with the maternal grandparents.

"I was taken from my husband's home and back to the home of my birth, for special care by my mother and father. The massage continues for a couple of months after birth. It is believed that, if the woman is given this special massage twice a day, then she will recover quickly and will be strong in the future."

Nutrient-rich in family

"In Nepalese society, all women have to work hard at their own home, which is why the new mother's parents take her back for the first three to four months after the baby's birth," says Samjhana. "It's a way to show their love and care for them.

"During my stay at my parents' home, my husband came to see the new baby from time to time," she recalls.

Her relatives also visited, with presents in hand – and no shortage of nutrient-filled food. She was frequently given *gudpak*, a

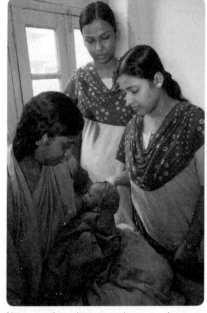

New mother learning how to breast-feed, India

Suckling to sleep

In the old Persian tradition, women are kept pampered and protected for forty days after giving birth. The newborn is tended to by the elder women of the family and handed over to the mother for regular breastfeedings. The mother is expected to eat healthy and nutritious foods, in order to give the baby hearty food through breast milk for those crucial first days.

The elder women busily prepare a variety of foods for the new mom:

Breakfast: *A creamy thick mixture of fresh cream and honey, warmed to perfection, along with lamb cooked so thoroughly as to be blended with a barley mixture, then sprinkled with cinnamon. This traditional rural breakfast is high in calories, as well as protein and dairy, to make the day's first full meal.*

Lunch: *Fresh vegetables and fruits of the season; in old Persia, these would be cut fresh from the fields for the new mom to consume endlessly. She would also be served a drink made from the seeds of grapes and quince, mixed with water and left overnight; by the next day, the water would turn syrupy and rich with nutrients.*

Dinner: *Skirt steak, cooked on an open fire, with the juices caught in a bowl beneath. The meat is consumed first, but the juices are not to be missed. The mother is then lulled to sleep with the juice of the meat, the baby suckling at her milk. Mom and baby are watched over until they fall asleep. A prayer is said over their heads each night and the same routine begins the next day.*

– *Maryam Zar, California, USA*

rich whole milk and cream dish with raisins, cardamom and other spices. Gifts for the baby included cloth, clothes and jewellery.

"By the time I returned to my husband's home, I had many gifts to bring with me, ranging from furniture from my maternal home and gold ornaments from the wealthier relatives to clothes, cash and other things for my daughter."

The art of breastfeeding

Breastfeeding is not an instinct; it is a learned skill, and, unless a woman has been shown or has seen how it is done, how is she to know how to position the baby at her breast? How is she to know that the fat-rich milk that provides the calories a baby needs comes at the end of the feed – and that the baby needs a good mouthful of breast as well as nipple to make this work?

The short stay in hospital for many modern mothers cuts into the time they need to establish their breastfeeding skills and gain the confidence to work through difficulties they may face as they continue breastfeeding at home. Not surprisingly, in cultures where women are fed and cared for by their own mothers and other female relatives for weeks after birth, with no other duties than to breastfeed the baby, it is rare to hear of mothers giving up after some weeks of struggle.

And it isn't just getting the baby to latch on well that can cause frustration – not to mention sore nipples and even mastitis. There are job responsibilities, care for older children and household chores to juggle, often without family support. Then there are social taboos around showing breasts and breastfeeding in public in some countries. Is it any wonder that new mothers sometimes struggle?

So what can help? Knowing that this is not easy, and all you can do is your best. Building a network of friends and supporters who can help you through and accepting any help that is on offer. Not blaming yourself if it doesn't work out as you hoped – and feeling okay with the choice to go to formula and a bottle if necessary. And giving yourself and the baby time you need to be together – and it will feel at times that feeding your newborn is a full-time occupation!

As with birth, what counts most now is love: the love that you and your baby are creating between you, whether breastfeeding or not.

All things pass. Pregnancy, birth and breastfeeding are part of the natural cycle of life. Live your life, love your babies, care for yourself, so that you can care for them too...And, oh yes, all things pass...
– *Cass McNamara, midwife*

Your meal is baby's meal

At a pregnant woman's baby shower, simple recipes are taught to her, with the focus on foods she needs to promote her breast milk. These are mainly traditional, like the different types of round beans, *nyimo*, *nyemba*, chick peas. Maize meal, not refined, will provide the staple, accompanied by these beans and beef. Dried vegetables called *mufuswa* cooked in *dovi* [peanut butter] are a speciality. *Mahewu*, a non-alcoholic drink, is popular; it is now commercially produced in different flavours.
– *Rebecca Pasipanodya, Zimbabwe*

A small nibble

The Dutch have a long history of providing home-based professional care for women and their families immediately after birth. This period is called the *kraamzorg*, literally translated as care during the lying-in period. A *kraamverzorgster*, or caregiver, assists the midwife during labour and stays with the family for the first eight days of the newborn's life. They keep watch on the health of both mother and baby, help first-time mothers learn how to care for an infant, take over the mother's household duties and care for any other children in the family, as well as guests who come to visit in those first few days.

Visitors are always welcomed by the *kraamverzorgster* with a warm cup of coffee and the traditional Dutch *beschuit en muisjes*, a round, toasted biscuit coated in anise seeds and sugar. The cookies have a little sugar tail, which is how they got their name – *muisjes* means mice. In the seventeenth century, around the time the biscuits first became popular, the anise seeds were believed to protect the mother and baby from evil spirits. Today, anise is known to stimulate breast-milk production.

During the *kraamzorg*, the new parents also receive a basket of gifts. This *kraammaandje* traditionally contains ten small presents for the mother, one to be opened each day, aimed at helping restore her well-being – things like scents and bath oils and brown beer (again, to stimulate breast-milk production). There are practical presents for the baby, including rompers, socks and toys. Fathers also now get a few presents to help them adjust to their new role, often a book on parenting or a bottle of beer.

– *Kathy Herschderfer, midwife, Netherlands*

Many soupy returns

Chicken is a common ingredient in recipes for new mothers around the world. In Eastern Europe, caraway seed soup with chicken is a popular variant suggested to those who are breast-feeding. Seeds such as caraway, anise, coriander, cumin and fennel are believed to naturally increase milk production, and they improve digestion.

Köménymag Leves
(Hungarian Caraway Seed Soup)

Ingredients

2 tbsp oil
1 tsp caraway seeds
2 tbsp flour
¼ tsp Hungarian paprika
4 cups chicken stock
salt to taste
croutons and/or sliced green onions to serve

Method

Place oil in a medium Dutch pot and add the caraway seeds. Sauté the seeds for 1 minute on low medium heat. Add the flour and keep stirring until flour begins to get a golden colour. Remove from heat and add the paprika. Gradually add the chicken stock and keep stirring until the flour is well blended with the stock. Taste and adjust the salt (the stock may have salt in it already). Bring soup to a slow simmer and simmer for 3 to 4 minutes. Remove from heat and cover pot. Let soup rest for 5 minutes. Serve piping hot with croutons and/or green onions.

In South Korea, expecting and new mothers eat *miyeok guk* (미역), or seaweed soup, during pregnancy and for the three weeks after birth. The seaweed used, *wakame* (sea mustard), is high in calcium and iodine, and the soup is believed to ensure nutritious breast milk and to help the mother towards recovery. Children are served the soup each year on their birthday to remind them of the pain and care their mother went through to bring them into the world!

Miyeok Guk (Seawood Soup)

Ingredients
1 cup dried *miyeok* (edible seaweed) — traditionally *wakame*, or sea mustard
16 cups water
7 oz (200 g) beef brisket, diced
1 tbsp minced garlic
4 to 5 tbsp fish sauce
sesame oil
rice

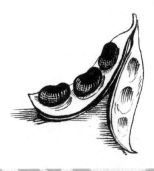

Method
Soak the *miyeok* in a bowl of water for at least 30 minutes. Drain and cut into bite-sized pieces. This should yield about 4 cups of rehydrated *miyeok*. In a stockpot, bring the *miyeok* and the water to a boil; keep at a boil at high heat for 20 minutes. If the broth becomes thick, add more water. Lower to medium heat and add the beef and garlic; simmer for 20 to 25 minutes. Add the fish sauce. Serve with a few spoonfuls of rice and a couple of drops of sesame oil.

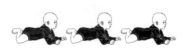

25

YOU "UGLY RAT":
NAMING NAMES (VIETNAM)

People all over the world do all they can to protect their new-borns from harm, wherever that might come from.

In Vietnam, for the first month of a child's life, she is considered especially vulnerable. During this period, babies are only visited by their closest relatives and are not officially named – it is said that an attractive name will entice evil spirits to come and "steal" the infant. Typical Vietnamese names are often highly compli-mentary, with meanings such as "lovely", "miracle", "gentle" and "peace", but, before the child reaches one month old, he is more likely to be called a repulsive name, such as "ugly", "rat" or even "shit". Once that critical first-month threshold has passed, the child is given his lasting name in a ceremony attended by the whole family.

Kiev Martin's mother, who is half Vietnamese, was opposed to celebrating the arrival of Kiev's new baby for fear of attract-ing misfortune. "We believe in waiting until thirty days after the birth for any celebrations," she says.

"In our tradition, we believe that the unborn child has a guardian angel, who is the previous mother of the child. If we celebrate the pregnancy publicly, the spirit of the previous parent might come and reclaim her child – so that the new mother loses her baby!"

As infant mortality has declined in Southeast Asia, the practice of calling your baby an "ugly rat" has become less fashionable, but some parents still prefer not to take the risk of giving the child her true name until she is safely beyond the reach of the spirit world.

A name, a place in history

The choice of a baby's name is hugely significant. Not only when that name is chosen, but also who chooses it, reflects the values and traditions of the larger community. In many cultures, a child's name symbolizes his links with past generations and the history of his people.

In Judaism, it is common to name a child after a family member who has recently died, in hopes that the child will emulate that person's virtues and keep her spirit alive. Yeshaya Adler, a graduate student at Rice University in Houston, Texas, explains the complex and extended family relationships and religious beliefs that lie behind the choices of names in his family.

"When I was born, my grandparents were both alive, so I wasn't named after anyone, but my younger siblings are named after my father's parents. My mother's mother passed away after we were born and named, so none of my siblings is named after her parents.

"My older brother is named after my father's older brother, Peter. But my father wanted to use a Hebrew name, so, because

Peter means 'rock' in Latin, he gave him the name Avniel, which means 'G-d is my rock'.

"After my father's father passed away, the next child born to him was a girl, so he gave my sister a middle name that started with the letter L, the first letter of his father's name. My next sibling was born after my father's mother passed away and he chose my grandmother's full initials to name my sister after her.

"Parents also reflect on the symbolic meaning of a name. For example, my first name, Yeshaya means 'G-d will save' or 'G-d is the savior'. 'Yah' means 'G-d is' or 'G-d will', so it's common to give a Jewish person a name that has this at the end, as with Yirmiyah (Jeremiah).

"A child's name is often picked well before it's born," Yeshaya says. "I've already given thought to what I will name my children. My girlfriend's grandfather has passed away, and so our first child that is male will be named after him."

History is also important. Yeshaya says that children's names frequently come from among the twelve tribes, prophets or leaders in Jewish history, or English, Greek or Latin rulers known to be particularly friendly to the Jewish people. "For example, Alexander the Great was known to be a friendly leader – he allowed Israel to remain autonomous – so Alexander is often given," he says.

A therapeutic name

The Jewish custom makes very clear that you do not name a child after someone who is living. "You wouldn't name your children after yourself as it's thought to draw the *ayin hara* (עָרה וְיע), the evil eye," says Yeshaya. "This is something that old Jewish grannies would worry about."

Names are powerful – so powerful that they may be called upon to heal a person through life. "A common matrilineal naming tradition involves healing. If you're sick, when your community prays for you, they pray for your name after your mother's name," he explains.

Furthermore, a person can gain a name to help with healing. "The middle name has a mystical purpose; in Hebrew tradition, if someone is very sick they might append a middle name to ask for healing. I have a friend who had cancer as a child and when he got sick his parents gave him the middle name Rafael, which means 'G-d will heal'. If the child gets well, they will either change or add another name to reflect that. Those names are added during religious services, so in a sense everyone is praying with you through those names."

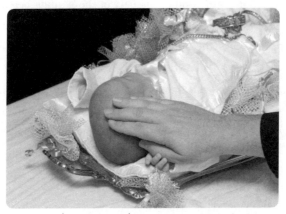

A *cohen* (Jewish priest) blesses a baby before his naming ceremony

Blessed identity

Yeshaya continues: "The name can be chosen any time up until the naming ceremony. There are different naming ceremonies for girls and boys, but both occur on the eighth day of the child's life.

"For boys, there is the *bris milah* (הְלִיֹמ תיִהְב), the circumcision ceremony – which is seen as a celebration with food and drinks to follow. For a girl's naming, the father will be called up to the Torah on the Saturday after the baby's birth to say a prayer, the *mi sheberakh* [a prayer of healing]. This prayer explains how G-d blessed the matriarchs [Sarah, Rebecca, Rachel, Leah, Miriam, Avigail, Devorah and Esther] and asks for blessings on this child as she is named and presented to the congregation."

Some Jewish families light a *ner nishamah* (רנ שמה), or "soul candle", as part of the naming ceremony. The candle, which burns for a day, memorializes the family members after whom the baby is named – it is the same type of candle used during mourning and at Yom Kippur, based on Proverbs 20:27, "The soul of man is a candle of the Lord." But, in this lighting of the candle, the parents also gratefully welcome the baby into the world.

Written on the body

In New Zealand, we have a variety of tattooing identities, such as the Pacifica and Maori patterns that are put on different parts of the body. These depict significant moments, like the passage to manhood, or when a person reaches a certain level of *mana*, or authority in the community based on relations with others.

I had been studying industrial design when we had our first child, Joshua. My wife, Paula, had helped me learn a bit of teeline shorthand to help record information from lectures. That was the inspiration. With a bit of design licence, we changed the proper placement of the shorthand symbols for our initials, so that when combined they looked balanced and well proportioned.

We created a teeline design that now incorporates all our first and second initials: MH (Matthew Harry), PM (Paula Maree), JH (Joshua Harry), OM (Olivia Margaret) and IG (Isaac George). As a teenager, I was in the scouting movement, so I decided that I would have the tattoo draped over my left shoulder, where senior scouts fix their braided cord. Paula has hers on the small of her back. Our children can continue the tattoo tradition if they wish, adding to it as they find a partner and eventually have children of their own.

What I really like is that we have started a new tradition of tattoo, which can grow and change with our family.

– *Matthew Wood, Wellington, New Zealand*

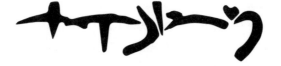

Matt and Paula's Maori-inspired teeline tattoo design

What's in a name?

A name has such a wealth of meaning that announcing one to the community calls for some very special ceremonies:

❖ A time for growth: At birth, a Maasai baby is given a "pet name", and, until the official name is bestowed on the child, the woman refrains from cutting her own hair – or the baby's. Then, when the child is given a proper name, the mother's and the child's head is shaved.

❖ A time for secrecy: In Japan, close family congregate seven days after the baby's birth for a formal naming ceremony called *oshichiya* (お七夜, or "seventh night"), which is the first big celebration for a baby in Japanese culture. Everyone else has to wait – including the local gods, who do not get to hear about the child's birth until the *omiyamairi*, the baby's first visit to a shrine.

❖ A time for celebration: The naming ceremony also takes place on the seventh day after birth in Ghana. "The husband gives the name to the child," says Georgina Nortey, who lives among the Ga people of Greater Accra. "The husband gives a fowl, drinks and money to prepare food for a get-together. The attire for the ceremony is white, but it is a very colourful event. There is music and dancing; a lot of people pay a visit to the mother and baby with gifts. It is a joyous occasion that cannot be forgotten."

❖ A time for security: An Inuit baby's name is traditionally chosen by the *angakkuq*, or shaman, who also decides on a protective spirit for the child. Children are often named after a recently deceased relative, with the idea that the baby will inherit that person's strengths. "It is okay to think of names, but our parents did not like us to name our children before they arrived in the world," says Julie Lys, a Métis nurse in the Northwest Territories, Canada.

❖ A time for good fortune: According to Lizzy Agams of Nigeria, "In Igboland, children are the most cherished possessions in every family, rich or poor. This is reflected in babies' names such as *Nwakaego*, meaning 'a child is greater than wealth'; *Amuruonyenaego*, meaning 'he who was born with money'; Egondu, meaning 'wealth of life'; *Egodikwa*, meaning 'there is wealth'."

"Be very careful"

Our daughter's naming ceremony, held when she was twelve days old, took place in New York City, not in India. Many of our friends came, and she was passed over and under the cradle three times, from woman to woman (with her male obstetrician muttering, "Be careful with that baby, I worked hard to get her here okay!"). Each of my five women friends whispered one of her names into her ear, after which we began to use her main name when speaking of or to her.

– Dr Saraswathy Ganapathy, Bangalore, India

Touched by the Earth

The Nepali Hindu eleventh-day naming ceremony is a lovely thing. At the first I attended, the naming part came very casually. The Brahmin just said, "Her name is Meg Kumari", and wrote it on a leaf in pink dye. We went outside, and he drew a chalk mandala in the center of the courtyard, made a little cup of dung in the middle and made offerings to it. He tied some string soaked in ghee to the baby's wrists, had the mother hold Meg Kumari over the *mandala* and pressed her tiny heel into the cup of dung: introducing the baby to the Sun, connecting her to the Earth.

My next naming ceremony was for the son of a Brahmin teacher who had shocked the village by marrying a Newar bride, a woman he'd met at university, breaking caste laws. I was proud of them for their courage and touched by their romance, and was the only guest at their sparse little Kathmandu apartment – they had left the village – for the baby's naming *puja*. On that occasion, the Brahmin determined that the first syllable of the baby's name should be "Bhu", and asked what name the parents wanted to choose that began with that sound. "Bhu, bhu," we all muttered, blanking on any name that started with "Bhu". I was the first to come up with a candidate: "Bhupendra?" I said tentatively. "Oh, yes!" his parents replied, and gave me the gift of naming their beautiful baby boy "king of the earth".
– *Paige Grant, New Mexico, USA*

26

AFARTANBAH: FORTY DAYS AND FORTY NIGHTS – OF REST (SOMALILAND)

Amy Szabo of Friends of Edna's Maternity Hospital has witnessed many births and their aftermath at Edna Adan University Hospital in Hargeisa, the capital of Somaliland. Among the women she remembers is Ayaan.

"Ayaan was surrounded by her mother, mother-in-law, sisters, neighbours and friends. The women were more than attentive, giving her water, feeding her spoonfuls of thin porridge, stroking her arm, holding her hand and walking beside her, stopping and embracing her whenever a labour pain came on," Amy says. "She was focused, able to find positions that were comfortable for her during contractions. When she dropped to her hands and knees, her sister brought a pillow for her to kneel on. When she was hot, three women started fanning her with the tails of their headscarves.

"In Somaliland, birth is a time for women to honour and support one another. Women are expected to be strong. The act of carrying and sustaining and nurturing and birthing describes so

Belly band

After birth, women in Liberia are given special herbal drinks to stimulate recovery, while leaves are woven together to make a special *lappa*, or body cloth, which is tied around her middle to keep her belly from wobbling too much.
— *Kathy Herschderfer, midwife, Netherlands*

much more of a woman's life than just the reality of pregnancy and childbirth. In this country of harsh landscapes and hard lives, birth is one time when a woman's strength is recognized and celebrated by those around her."

A break from it all

Seven days after she gave birth to Muna, Ayaan's close family held a naming ceremony. But, in order to ward off illness and evil spirits, Muna's extended family did not get to meet her for another forty days, a period commemorated with a big celebration known as *afartanbah* (ةبنطرف) – "the exit from confinement". For those forty days, Ayaan and Muna stayed indoors, rested, bonded and healed. Close female relatives took great care of them both, ensuring they followed local traditions to keep them safe, such as wearing earrings made of garlic to ward off the "evil eye".

Amy goes on: "Traditionally, the husband will move out of the house during those forty days. In the countryside, the family builds a small hut or tent beside the main house for him to live in. In the city, the husband moves in with other family, or stays in the same house but doesn't share the bed. The essential tradition is that the husband and wife do not have sexual relations until forty days after *afartanbah*, and the celebration is treated almost like a mini-wedding.

"After forty days of rest, Muna was strong and growing and Ayaan was healed enough to resume her responsibilities in the household as wife and mother. Ayaan wore her best dress and looked beautiful for the party, and as she welcomed her husband back into their home."

Ayaan and Muna were lucky to be attended by a trained midwife at the hospital; only nine percent of women in Somaliland get a chance to give birth with a skilled attendant. Edna Adan University Hospital, which was founded by Edna Adan Ismail – a native of Somaliland who trained as a midwife in the UK and later became first lady and a UN diplomat – was one of the first facilities to offer safe, clean and modern maternity care after the country's civil war.

A time to heal

Language says a great deal about our thinking around childbirth. Nurse-midwife Jody Lori points out that "confinement" has been used to refer to the "lying-in" period just after birth for centuries, but being "confined" – detained or, worse, imprisoned – can make a new mother feel completely alone during this difficult transition.

A similar term, *la cuarentena* ("the quarantine"), is used to describe the forty-day period after birth when women in Latin

Waiting time

We are given a special beef bone soup to make us strong. We have tea in a Thermos next to us all the time so we can drink it whenever we want. You have to wear a tight binder around your stomach and keep your legs crossed when you sit and lie down, otherwise air can go in when you talk or laugh.

After some time, about a week, the women church members and friends come with gifts and pray or sing hymns. Then the baby and mother can go outdoors. We massage the baby with oil with special herbs — I know what they look like, but I don't know the name. After that, I rested for another month; my mother-in-law came and did all the housework during this time.

A woman's own mother has to wait to be invited to see the baby, and she has to come with presents for the baby — clothes, soap, oil, towels. She also brings presents for the new mother and the mother-in-law.

— *Afande Jephrace and Esther Sikote, Luiya people, Kenya, in conversation with the Belaku Trust*

America rest. During this time, they are supposed to consume lots of chicken soup and carrots — but avoid spicy food. They wrap the tummy with a cotton or muslin cloth called a *faja* to aid in healing. They are also supposed to focus on bonding with their newborns. The tradition is believed to have biblical roots, based on the forty days prescribed for cleansing the woman after giving birth in Leviticus 12:1–5.

In Karnataka, southern India, the months after *herige*, or childbirth, involve a series of special customs called *banānthānā* (बनांथाना),

the closest translation into English being the old-fashioned concept of "confinement". It is a time of rest and recuperation for the mother and her womb (*karalu*), during which she is cared for by other women. She is given special foods and is exempt from all housework. The aim is to safeguard the baby's health, by preserving the mother's health and well-being now and far into the future.

As older women in Karnataka put it, the new mother, known as the *bananthi*, has a *hasi mayi* – a "tender body". According to Dr Saraswathy Ganapathy of the Belaku Trust, women often say, "If we do not do a strict *banānthānā*, the mother will be weak in later life."

"Like a sucked-out mango stone"

Banānthānā grows out of the belief that pregnancy is a time when "bad fluids" accumulate in the body. The older women of the community can be quite vocal about the need to cleanse the body. They will be heard saying, "A *bananthi* should become thinner than she was before pregnancy. She should become like the tip of *mantani* leaf – thin, tender, fresh and supple."

"She must become like a sucked-out mango stone, like a sliver of *chakke* [wood]."

"She must become *sundu hippe* – dried and desiccated."

"All the bad water should be drained from the body."

Eating particular foods, considered to be "hot" in the ayurvedic system of medicine, is essential for eliminating the "bad" fluids. "Ideally a *bananthi* loses these fluids in a three-month period and becomes 'half her size'," explains Saras. "A new mother's *karalu* is *hasi* [tender], as well as inflamed and loose. She should therefore eat only small quantities of bland food. The food that a

Brought into the fold

In our Nepalese mythology, there are four castes or classes of people: *brahmins* (priest class); *kshtriya* (warrior class); *vaishya* (farmers and business people); and *sudra* (servants and labouring class). It is believed that the newborn infant is still impure, or an "outcast" (with no class), until the ritual of *nwaran* is performed on the eleventh day after birth. This is because the baby has been in-side the mother's body, which is considered "impure"; *nwaran* is the sacred ritual to purify the baby and to accept her into the father's caste. It is essential as part of this ritual to record the time, month and year of the baby's birth according to the Hindu calendar.

Nwaran is also the occasion for naming the baby. The family priest, a *brahmin*, performs all the rituals. All the male and female deities are named and honoured prior to the naming of the infant. Then, the infant is accepted into the caste and provided with a surname and a *nwaran* name, which denotes the child's horoscope for the rest of her life.

It is also customary that the mother and infant are not touched by any male members of the family – including the baby's father – until this eleventh day. As a new mother, I was kept in a separate room with my baby and not allowed to be near my husband until this purifying ritual; I found that very difficult. I was a new daughter-in-law, after only fourteen months of marriage, so I was unused to speaking up for my needs in front of my mother-in-law and other family. Although my husband had always been by my side, it was not easy for him to help me in our traditional family, where a son is not supposed to help his wife. As I was weak from the birth, tired from lack of sleep and had little knowledge of breastfeeding, I found the cultural dos and don'ts quite frustrating!

– *Samjhana Phuyal, Kathmandu, Nepal*

mother eats is also seen to affect her breast milk. If a breastfeeding mother eats 'cold' or 'gas-producing' foods, it is said the baby
will be prone to problems such as colic or diarrhoea."

Women strongly believe that "cold" elements in the ayurvedic
system of medicine must be prevented from entering the body in
any way, and so they are encouraged to lie down and keep their
legs crossed. One first-time mother called Sunita put it like this:
"A *bananthi* should rest and lie down all of the time. She should
not sit for any length of time because, although she may not feel
the pain now, she is sure to feel pain in fifty years' time."

In the weeks after childbirth, the mother is at risk from *drishti* –
possession by spirits, which cause illnesses. Saras goes on: "*Banānthānā*
is seen as the best protection the community can provide for mother
and baby alike.

"New mothers may find it hard to follow the rules of *banānthānā*,
especially when they become thirsty, but traditionally they believe
it is good for them and for the baby and so they do their best to
comply." For this reason, when families can afford it, the care and
rest of *banānthānā* may be extended from three months up to seven.

✳ ✳ ✳ ✳ ✳ ✳ ✳ ✳ ✳ ✳ ✳ ✳ ✳ ✳

The four stages of bananthana

"*Banānthānā* is divided into four stages, each marked by rituals and changes in diet and activity.

From birth to day 3, mother and child are confined to a dark room, where they are kept warm and only visited by family and other caregivers. Twice a day, the mother is given foods like *rava ganji* with *jaggery* (a thin semolina porridge with unrefined sugar), or coffee with *jaggery*. She must drink hot water, and only after meals. She is also given betel leaf and betel nut with lime (a mild stimulant), for chewing. The mother must lie down and do no work, and a cloth binder is tied around her to support her back and belly.

On or near day 3, *meen* and turmeric paste are smeared on the mother's body; then she is given a bath and her hair is washed and dried with *samrani* (incense). It is a common belief that the breast milk descends after this ritual, and so this is the time to begin breastfeeding. Her diet is bland – just rice and salt.

From day 11 to day 40, the mother is given a shot of *arrack* (a drink often made from fermented coconut flower sap) or brandy after a "head bath" to ward off "cold" elements. The time of ritual seclusion is ended. The house is cleansed and new pots are brought in. She is given "hot" foods and flavourings – chicken, goat meat, dried prawns, pepper, garlic and cumin – and just a few green vegetables. She must still avoid "cold" vegetables, *utcche yellu* (sesame seed oil) and cold water. Ideally, she remains exempt from work, although where a family does not have much money, this may not be possible.

From day 40 to the third or fourth month, the mother may visit the temple, or leave the house with her child for essential visits. Her "confinement" is nearly over, and she may start eating foods like *ragi* (millet balls). And, if she comes from an affluent household, she continues to rest as much as possible!

– *Dr Saraswathy Ganapathy, Asha Kilaru, Zoe Matthews, Jayashree Ramakrishna and Shanti Mahendra, Belaku Trust*

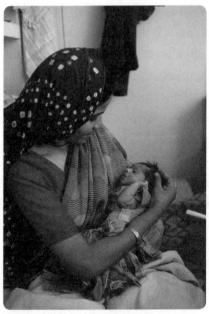

Mother and baby, India

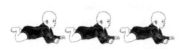

27

"SHE HAS JUST GIVEN BIRTH!" (TANZANIA)

When my first child was born, I remember how people would call out '*Nawore mfee!*' when they saw my husband and me," recalls Rose Mlay, who is from the Kilimanjaro region of northern Tanzania. "In our language this means 'She has just given birth to a baby', and it signifies that people must give priority to the woman and her family, and show empathy towards the new mother."

> This is how my tribe makes sure that new mothers are loved and cared for.
> – Rose Mlay, Chagga people, Tanzania

"As a new mother, I was not supposed to do anything except eat, breastfeed and sleep, day or night, for four months after my babies were born. My husband – like all husbands in our region – was expected to save enough money to make sure I could give birth at the health centre (rather than at home without help from a trained midwife, as too many women do). Like all husbands, he also saved up so that as a new mother I could eat nutritious foods, in particular meat and milk."

The work of a new father

"If a man has no mother, sisters or sisters-in-law living nearby, he has to do all the housekeeping work," Rose explains. "My husband was a medical intern at the time, so he was very busy, but we had no family near so he did all the shopping and cooking for me. Men in Tanzania rarely cook except for this occasion, and he made me a big pot of food – beef and bananas. When he came home and saw I hadn't eaten it, he worried that it was because he was not a good cook, but, really, I only felt like drinking tea. It was funny!

"The husbands of new mothers make a lot of effort to look after them. If there is no form of transport, they may walk for five kilometres or more, carrying a twenty-litre bucket of milk on their heads – and they have to do this every weekend.

"But the man also gets special consideration because of the community's respect for the new mother. When the father of a new baby goes shopping for food for his wife, the other shoppers and shopkeepers (mostly men) will make way for him, telling each other, '*Nawore mfee!*' The butcher will also give him the best meat cuts, every day, because the people all know that the new mother needs to eat food containing either meat or milk each day."

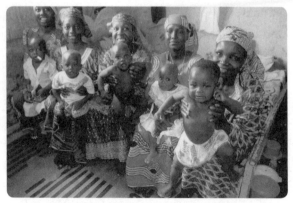

New mothers showing off their babies

Plenty for everyone

Rose goes on: "Pregnant women are really cherished and now they are taken to give birth at health facilities. From the time I grew up in my village, Mwika Maringa, until today, I have not heard of a single woman who died in childbirth.

"Chagga women work very hard for their households when they are not pregnant, but, as soon as they are new mothers, they are assured of peace and rest for these four months. In fact, they gain weight – sometimes too much – as it is not acceptable for them to lack anything they need. When we were children, we always used to visit the houses of neighbours who had babies as there was a very happy atmosphere and plenty of food for everyone!

"When I was a little girl, I overheard my father advising my brother, who did not like cooking, that he must learn how to cook because, when he gets married and his wife gives birth, it will be his responsibility."

A new metric

Just at this moment when you could really do with a good long sleep, it becomes impossible. Your newborn doesn't know the difference between night and day and isn't aware of the concept of "bedtime" – and probably won't be for months to come. And, if you already have children, their demands on you are likely to be more, not less, as they come to terms with the arrival of a tiny, wrinkled and often wailing creature into the middle of their family.

Arianna Huffington, the editor-in-chief of *Huffington Post*, recently launched the "Third Metric" project to reassess the ways we define success in life. "Our national delusion that the way to be ultra-productive is to cut back on sleep is particularly destructive for women," she says.

"On average, single working women and working mothers actually get an hour and a half less sleep than the seven-and-a-half-hour minimum the body needs to function. Which, really, is no surprise. Just because women have added responsibilities in the workplace doesn't mean the division of labor at home has changed accordingly. And, in the macho boys' club atmosphere that dominates many offices, women too often feel they have to overcompensate by working harder, longer and later."

Arianna speaks from personal experience. "In 2007, sleep-deprived and exhausted, I fainted, hit my head on my desk, broke my cheekbone and got four stitches above my right eye. And, even as it's affecting our health, sleep deprivation will also profoundly affect your creativity, your productivity and your decision-making. The Exxon Valdez wreck, the explosion of the

Challenger space shuttle and the nuclear accidents at Chernobyl and Three Mile Island – all were at least partially the result of decisions made on too little sleep."

So treat your tiredness with respect; it is telling you something. It means don't expect too much of yourself, take it as easy as you can, and above all ask for help and accept it.

One sleep potion

In Moldova, when a child is born, the family traditionally hosts a celebration to which all the older women of the family are invited. The women relatives bring food and other gifts for the mother and newborn and prepare baths for them.

Before her bath, the woman is massaged with oil infused with myrrh. Afterwards, she drinks a mix of wine and herbs to ease her way to the sleep she so needs for recovery.

The child is also bathed by the older women of the family – in holy water spiked with honey and herbs. Symbolic items are placed in the bathing water: an apple (representing fertility); an item of gold (so the child will grow up to be rich); coins (so the child will know how to deal with money); a watch (so the child will know how to keep track of time); and a book (so the child will be clever).

The older women then take care of the baby and all household duties while the mother sleeps. And, while she sleeps, they celebrate the birth of the baby with food and wine.

Plenty of rest

Getting enough rest in the early days may seem impossible, but sleep is essential for coping with the stress of a newborn and enjoying your new family. Some tips:

- ❖ Sleep when your baby sleeps; leave the housework for another time!
- ❖ If you are not getting enough sleep by sleeping when your child sleeps, ask a relative or friend to take care of your baby – and use that time to rest.
- ❖ Most new mothers find it hard to stay awake, but if you get seriously overtired you can also find it hard to drop off to sleep – so do something relaxing for half an hour before you go to bed, like soaking in a warm bath.
- ❖ Try a form of meditation called "deep relaxation". Get as comfortable as possible – sitting or lying down – and close your eyes. Breathe in deeply and slowly and quietly through your nose. Let each breath out slowly through your mouth. Tense the muscles of your left leg as much as you can and then release the tension – let it all go loose. Do the same with your right leg, each arm, your neck and head, and your chest. Then imagine your body becoming very heavy, sinking into the ground beneath you. Slowly resume your normal breathing pace and open your eyes – if you can. (You can learn about deep relaxation exercises online.)

28

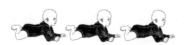

NAKI! NAKI! NAKI!: SUMO-WEIGHT SOOTHING (JAPAN)

Some days (or nights), it may seem impossible to soothe your baby to sleep. But there may be some lessons to be gained from enterprising Japanese parents who escort their infants to Sensoji Temple in Hiroshima each spring for the *Nakizumo* festival, which is held on Children's Day. *Nakizumo* (泣き相撲) literally translates as "crying baby sumo", and at the festival parents hope to *make* their baby cry before anyone else's.

The festival seems quite conventional in many ways. Parents dress their baby in a *kimono*, the traditional robe. At the *dohyō*, or sumo ring, the child is placed on a cushion facing his competitor. Then, to get things started, a student sumo wrestler holds each baby in the air, shouting, "*Naki! Naki! Naki!*" ("Cry! Cry! Cry!").

If this doesn't actually start off a fit of wailing, the wrestler then makes frightening faces and noises. If this doesn't do the trick, an *oni*, or ogre, mask is donned by the *gyoji*, or referee. The first child to start crying is often named the winner – and, if there's a draw, the prize goes to the longest crying or loudest baby.

The roots of this festival lie in a Japanese proverb, *Naku ko wa sodatsu* ("Crying babies grow fast"). The competition is meant to encourage the growth of a physically and spiritually robust baby – and, in the days of high infant mortality, a crying baby was considered to be healthy enough to alert her parents that she needed attention. The sounds of all the babies' cries are also supposed to drive away any lingering malevolent spirits. Parents pray for their child's health throughout the competition.

Babies don't always co-operate, however; some of them do manage to sleep or laugh through the whole ordeal!

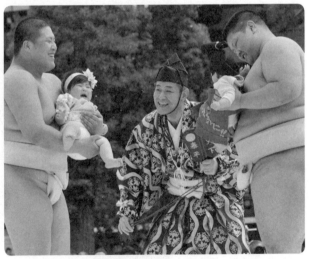

Babies and wrestlers face off in the *dohyō*

✳ ✳ ✳ ✳ ✳ ✳ ✳ ✳ ✳ ✳ ✳ ✳ ✳ ✳

Laughing through the hard times

I have four children and could bang on *forever* about the joys, perils, nightmares, fears, ecstasies, terrors, lone-liness, passions and spirituality of the baby days. But other people wanted to write in this book too...so I would love you to remember me for just *one* thing, the greatest post-childbirth tip and the biggest gift I can bestow.

After you've given birth, whether you've had stitches or not, the prospect of the "Stinging Wee" looms large.

Fear no longer. When you need to go – run a few inches of water in the bath. Get in and wee there. As you're reading this, you may be thinking, "Meh, what's the big deal there?"

But, dear expectant or new mother, when it happens, you will be shouting my name from the rooftops, in a good way.

May you always remember me as the person who stopped your front bottom from smarting.

– *Emma Freud, writer, broadcaster, contributor to Comic Relief and White Ribbon Alliance Champion*

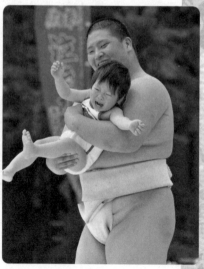

At the *Nakizumo* festival

From "Cradle Song"

Sleep, sleep, beauty bright,
Dreaming in the joys of night;
Sleep, sleep; in thy sleep
Little sorrows sit and weep.

Sweet babe, in thy face
Soft desires I can trace,
Secret joys and secret smiles,
Little pretty infant wiles.

As thy softest limbs I feel,
Smiles as of the morning steal
O'er thy cheek, and o'er thy breast
Where thy little heart doth rest.

O the cunning wiles that creep
In thy little heart asleep!
When thy little heart doth wake,
Then the dreadful night shall break.

– *William Blake (1757–1827)*

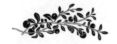

Time for cradle songs

Rhythm, rocking, singing – these things are universally soothing, no matter what your age. So of course, mothers everywhere sing to their babies.

And now scientists have come up with evidence for what
mothers have always known: according to researchers at Great
Ormond Street Hospital in London, lullabies do not merely
calm babies and young children, but lower their heart rate and
reduce their perception of pain. The best remedies are often of
our own making.

Dorme Nênem (Brazil)

Dorme nênem que a cuca vai pegar,
Mamãe foi para roça e papai foi trabalhar.

Sleep, Baby

Sleep baby, or the dragon will come to get you,
Mum's gone to the field and dad's gone to work.
– André Simões

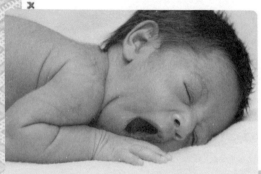

Sleep, baby

东北摇篮曲 *(China)*
月儿明 风儿静
树叶挂窗棂
小宝宝 快睡觉
睡在那个梦中

月哪个明 风儿哪个静
摇篮轻拍动
娘的宝宝闭上眼睛
睡呀睡在那个梦中

Northeastern Cradle Song

The moon is bright, the wind is quiet,
The tree leaves hang over the window,
My little baby, go to sleep quickly,
Sleep, dreaming sweet dreams.

The moon is bright, the wind is quiet,
The cradle moving softly,
My little one, close your eyes,
Sleep, sleep, dreaming sweet dreams.

Los Pollitos (Argentina)

Los pollitos dicen pío, pío, pío

Cuando tienen hambre

Cuando tienen frío.

La gallina busca el maíz y el trigo

Les da la comida y les presta abrigo.

Bajo sus dos alas, acurrucaditos

¡Duermen los pollitos

Hasta el otro día!

La gallina dice cloc, cloc, cloc

Cuando canta el gallo

Cuando sale el sol

The Little Chicks

The little chicks say peep, peep, peep

When they're hungry

And when they're cold

The hen looks for corn and wheat

Gives them food and keeps them warm

Under her two wings, curled up

Sleep, chicks,

Until another day!

The hen says cluck, cluck, cluk

When the rooster sings

And the sun comes out

Ghumparani, mashi pishi (Bengali)

Ghumparani, mashi pishi
Moder bari esho,
Khat debo palong debo
Chouki pete bosho.
Bata bhore paan debo
Gaal bhore kheyo,
Khukur chokheh ghum nai
Ghum diye jeyo

Aunties, Aunties, Bring Us Sleep

Aunties, aunties, bring us sleep,
Visit our home,
We'll bring you the cot along with the bedding,
For now sit on a chair.
We'll give you the *paan* (betel leaf) container, have your fill
To chew and enjoy as you stuff it in your cheek,
For now the Little One has no sleep in her eyes
Give her some before you leave.

– Gouri Guha, India

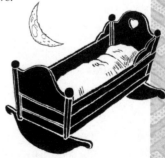

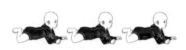

29

A MOTHER'S TOUCH:
WEARING THE *KANGA* (EAST AFRICA)

They are found throughout East Africa, particularly in Tanzania and Kenya: boldly and brightly printed rectangles of durable cotton known as *kangas*. Indeed, there is a saying in Swahili: a woman cannot be happy until she has had a thousand *kangas*. Of course, not all *kangas* are used for carrying babies. They can be worn as skirts, sleeping wear or kitchen aprons, among other things.

"I was born in Dar es Salaam; therefore, *kangas* have 'raised me'," says Chiku Lweno-Aboud, who works in Tanzania for the Mama Ye! campaign. "These pieces of cloth are used to wrap newborns immediately after birth, and eventually are used to tie babies and toddlers on their mother's back."

Beginning sometime early in the twentieth century, Swahili proverbs were added to the basic design. This writing is called the *jina* (name) or *ujumbe* (message). It is said that the *ujumbe* was first added by a trader based in Mombasa, perhaps in an attempt to get a leg up on his competition. The artwork also carries a meaning. "The coastal Swahili culture is rich in expressions, and these have been creatively captured in *kanga* messages for years," says Chiku. "When I see one in a shop, or someone passes by wearing a *kanga*, my eye automatically moves to the strapline at the bottom to read what it says!"

In most cases, the *kanga*'s use will depend on what it has to say for itself. Many *kangas* are given as gifts – the equivalent of a greeting card. Chiku continues: "I have given *kangas* as condolences, as wedding presents, as gifts for other special days. The beauty of a *kanga* is that it 'speaks' for you. It is a clothing that encourages creativity – Swahili women have many ways of tying *kangas*. They can be used for wearing a baby, swaddled around an infant, tied like a sarong, wrapped around the waist or thrown carefully over the mother and the baby's heads like a loose veil."

They make a great, practical gift for a new mother – a time-tested means for carrying a child close to the body.

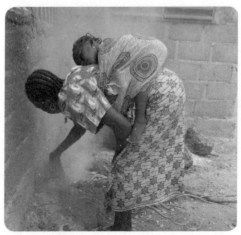

Mother carrying baby with *kanga*, Burkina Faso

How to tie a *kanga*

1) Hold the *kanga* stretched out behind you, with the top edge at your waist.

2) While keeping hold of the *kanga*, lean forward and have someone cradle the baby onto your back, facing you, with its bottom in line with your waist.

3) Slide the *kanga* upwards, towards your shoulders, catching and covering the baby's bottom to hold her on your back, but keeping her legs free.

4) Take the right edge of the *kanga* and pull it over your right shoulder.

5) Pull the left edge of the *kanga* under your left arm.

6) Tie together the ends fast and snug at your chest.

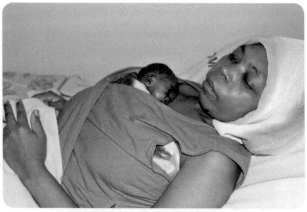

Mother providing "kangaroo care", Rwanda

Kangaroo care

"Wearing a baby" *kanga*-style brings many benefits – especially for a baby who feels safe and contented on his parent's back or chest.

A similar but unrelated care method, called "kangaroo mother care", involves placing a baby in skin-to-skin contact on the mother's or father's chest for hours at a time. The practice got its name from the way a kangaroo mother carries her newborn joey in the pouch. Pre-term infants are often nurtured in this manner, soothing the baby, keeping her at the right temperature, boosting breastfeeding and reducing the newborn's sensitivity to any painful medical interventions. And, in countries where intensive-care baby units are simply not available, kangaroo care has proved to be a life-saver.

When Omari Ali was told that his newborn twins were severely underweight at 1.5 kilograms (3 pounds, 5 ounces) and needed kangaroo care, he was worried that even swaddling his fragile-looking babies close to his body might hurt them in some way. His nervousness disappeared with the patient and encouraging coaching of Mama Ye! nurses in Tanzania, who emphasized the benefits of sharing with his wife the daily work of nurturing the babies.

"You feel very warm, but that's how it should be, as the child feels as if he was in his mother's womb," explains Ali. "I would hold the child in this position for about two hours, then I take him to his mother for breastfeeding."

He arranged to leave work three times a day to partner with his wife, Salma Issa, in this critical care for their babies.

Finding the message

When choosing a *kanga* for baby-carrying, consider these *ujumbe*:

Mama nibariki mungu anizidishie
Mama bless me and God multiply the blessings
Decoding: *Mungu* means "God"

Uchungu wa mwana aujuae mzazi
The pain of a child is known by the parent
One meaning: Whether the pain of childbirth or the pain of a
   child growing up, a parent always knows the child best

Mtoto umleavyo ndivyo akuavyo
The way you raise your children determines what they will grow / be
Decoding: *Mtoto* means "child"

Kazi mwanamandanda, kulala njaa kupenda
Work is an obedient child; sleeping hungry is one's choice
Decoding: The root *-lala* means "to sleep"; *-lala fofofo* means to
   sleep like a log!

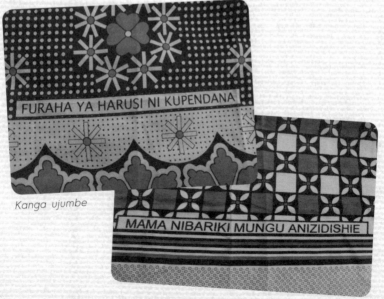

Kanga ujumbe

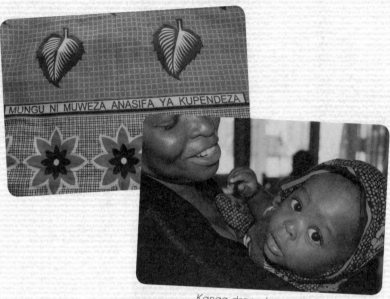

Kanga draped over baby, Tanzania

Penzi la mama tamu, haliishi hamu
Sweet mother's love – desire for it never dies
Meaning: A mother's love is so sweet, you never have enough of it

Ufunguo wa heri ni baraka
The key to happiness and blessings
Decoding: Usually illustrated with a pineapple or other sweet fruit, to represent love, beauty, or a good upbringing (and sometimes even conjugal bliss!)

Titi la mama ni tamu
The mother's milk is the best

Ni chumu
Good luck!
One meaning: On a *kanga*, saying *Ni chumu* so boldly means more than "good luck", and should be read as "Look at me, it's good luck, all that I have" or "Life is fate, you can't predict how it will go".

✖✖✖✖✖✖✖✖✖✖✖✖✖

30

GOING HOT AND COLD: *ZUOYUEZI* (CHINA)

After giving birth, Chinese mothers follow *zuoyuezi* ("doing the month", 坐月子). During this time, they must rest, a social rule that helps to ensure recovery from labour and delivery. They avoid going outside and bathing, which protects both mother and baby from exposure to infection. And they should eat hearty, healthy "hot" fare – meaning food classified as "hot", or *yang*, in the balance of forces known as *yinyang* (陰陽).

Foods are considered "hot" or "cold" based on whether they induce heat or coldness in the body, according to traditional Chinese medicine. During pregnancy, women are encouraged to eat "cold" foods, but, during labour and after childbirth, the menu turns "hot". "Hot" foods include chicken soup with sesame oil, hard-boiled eggs, papaya (*paw paw*), pineapple, fermented tapioca or rice, sugarcane juice, ginger, garlic (in moderation), bamboo shoot, cooked dark leafy greens, cooked carrots, and rice wine and other alcohol. If an expecting or new mother breaks the rules of *yinyang*, it is said that she puts herself at risk of miscarriage, difficult birth and illness.

"Doing the month" has been recorded since at least the Song dynasty (960–1279), and about seventy percent of new mothers observe the month-long period at the home of their mother-in-law (or mother), who is considered the expert in all things *zuoyuezi* – a post-birth rule that helps to build the bonds of the extended family. Some modern hospitals have set up *zuoyuezi* centres to care for new mothers and babies who are far from their extended family in those first weeks after birth, or a *yuepo* (confinement nanny) can be hired to help out at home.

But not all of the old ways are still followed. For instance, many women choose not to add "hot" beer or rice wine to their soup to improve circulation, since it can have a detrimental effect on a developing or breastfeeding baby, unless they boil off all the alcohol. And bathing is usually considered a good thing, despite the "cold" yin of plain water!

Sauna time

"All went well with my baby's birth, and right afterwards my parents came to live with me to look after me," remembers Kiev Martin, whose father is Chinese and whose mother is half Chinese. "In Asian culture, you have to lie on your back in bed, breastfeeding while your mother or your sister takes care of you, and takes the baby to be changed and bathed."

> In traditional Chinese medicine, the mother's body needs heat – in many forms – to recover from the birth.
> – *Kiev Martin, Maryland, USA*

"Every day for a month after the birth, my dad got up at four every morning. His job was to heat up a stone of about ten pounds in weight, which he found on a construction site. He did this in a gas stove in the garage for about an hour until it was very hot. Then the stone was wrapped in towels and brought to me to be placed on my belly for about four or five hours. This was meant to reduce the swelling in my abdomen after the birth, and reduce the stress caused by birth. It was pretty comforting and did reduce the size of my belly quite quickly."

For Kiev, that meant a daily sauna. Kiev continues: "They really like you to sweat to purify your body through your pores, and I had to keep warm and warmly dressed all the time. The tradition is to create a kind of sauna, with a bowl of boiling water with lemon leaves next to the woman and a blanket over her and the steaming bowl. The only part of the mother you can see is her face!"

This is a common practice in Cambodia, where midwife Theresa Shaver also recalls coals being placed under a new mother's bamboo bed to warm the room in a tradition called *sor sai kjey*.

"Heat was also applied through a menthol body rub," says Kiev. "Every morning my mom would massage my body from head to toe with a mint preparation called Ricqlès, which she ordered from Paris." (Ricqlès is now sold as a soft drink, but it is still available as a medicinal spirit.)

And, of course, "hot" foods were served. "Before breakfast, my mother would bring me a shot of alcohol to drink – usually rum or whisky," Kiev remembers. "Normally, I don't drink so I did find this a hard challenge! In Asian culture, we believe that this heats up our internal system, and avoids incontinence when we are older. She also made me three fresh meals a day with foods with a lot of 'heat' in them, including ginger and black pepper (but not chilli). For breakfast every day, she made me *congee* [a rice porridge] with stir-fried pork and ginger. I was not supposed to eat any 'cooling foods', such as salad or raw vegetables."

Old and new

For Kiev, who lives in Maryland and works for the American College of Nurse Midwives, it wasn't always easy. "I found it hard to comply with all this in the USA, but I did try," she says. "I didn't leave my room for the first three weeks and I was a bit bored and lonely. People are allowed to visit you, but not for long, as the fear is that you will develop spider veins if you walk around, or a bad back if you sit up.

"My in-laws came to visit me and the baby, and they were expected to contribute to the chores as I was not supposed to clear up after them or do any housework. My American mother-in-law was very progressive, so she was back at work within hours of the birth of her son, so it must have seemed strange to them.

"With my second baby, I did not comply as much with the routine, because I needed to work. In fact, I was still taking phone calls when I went to the hospital, and I did work on the phone from my bed when I got home. But my mother was not happy with me about that. And I do think the traditional system worked better for me; I recovered better the first time around."

✺ ✺ ✺ ✺ ✺ ✺ ✺ ✺ ✺ ✺ ✺ ✺ ✺ ✺ ✺

Closing the bones

Many doulas, such as Stacia Smales Hill (doula.org.uk) in the UK and Pam England in the USA (birthingfromwithin.com), connect the experience of birth to the story of Inanna, told on a four-thousand-year-old Sumerian clay tablet that is thought to be the first written myth. In the story, Inanna takes a perilous journey down into the Underworld, losing her life in the process. It is her twin sister who has killed her. But spirits that have come to rescue Inanna hear the sister in the agony of labour and support her. In gratitude, Inanna's twin breathes life back into her sister who escapes from the Underworld and returns to the world of the living. "This is what happens in birth, as in so many other times of a woman's life," says Stacia. "When we have a baby, part of us dies, and we are reborn as a mother. The essential male myth is that of going out to slay dragons; the essential and oldest women's myth is that of death and rebirth, over and over again."

The Mexican *rebozo* shawl is used in a ritual to mark this death and rebirth of the woman. "During birth, a woman is stripped, open, exposed as never before," Stacia explains, "and it takes time for her to physically come together again. She also needs to come together again emotionally."

Doulas like Stacia practise a ritual based on the Mexican tradition of "closing the bones". "We make the new mother warm, give her a bath with herbal infusions – a *baño de hier-*

bas – and wrap her from head to toe in the *rebozo*, so that she feels swaddled and squeezed and hugged. I have seen women cry from the emotion of feeling so much 'wrapped in love'," Stacia says. The herbs in the bath can help restore the mother's warmth, increase her milk flow and blood circulation, soothe tired muscles and promote relaxation.

Afterwards, the mother is laid in the *rebozo* and her women attendants literally "hug" her body back together, healing her, mind, body and spirit.

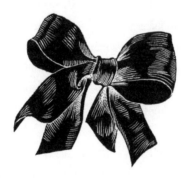

A doctor's view on going hot and cold

The body is very good at maintaining its optimal temperature – around 37 degrees Celsius (98.6 degrees Fahrenheit). Heating the body seems to cause a reflex reaction through which blood moves from the deeper tissues to the surface in order to cool down.

During the second and third trimester of pregnancy, the womb is engorged with blood. During the birth of the baby and the delivery of the placenta, some blood vessels are damaged, and the less blood in an area, the less chance of haemorrhage. By pulling the blood to the body's surface, humans have throughout evolution reduced the risk of excessive bleeding.

In addition, the process of birth triggers adrenaline and other "fight or flight" hormones and neurotransmitters. These prompt cell activity that generates waste products, some of which are potentially damaging free radicals. Sweating will help remove these.

Alcohol and spicy foods cause what is known as peripheral blood vessel dilation – opening up skin capillaries and moving blood from inner organs and tissues to the surface for cooling. Hot food and drinks also encourage sweating. Sweat as it evaporates removes heat from the body, but it also has the added benefit of detoxifying the tissues. This is because water-soluble toxins are released through the sweat.

Similarly, massage has a mild bruising effect and heats the skin, again pulling blood away from internal organs.

Isolation after birth reduces the risk of infection from others. Lying down for long periods of time removes the gravitational effect of blood loss from the uterus, and also reduces the risk of uterine and bladder prolapse. Rest also allows the strained ligaments and tendons that hold the bones and muscles of the pelvis to realign and strengthen; this helps prevent lower back problems in the long term.

Resting the mother, cleaning the house, providing fresh food and ensuring the antiseptic benefits of spicy foods (particularly garlic and turmeric) all help prevent infectious disease.

– Dr Rajendra Sharma MB BCh BAO LRCP&S (Ire) MFHom, integrated physician and author of Live Longer, Live Younger

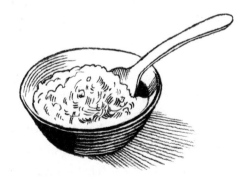

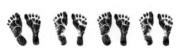

31

THE CHAIN OF GODMOTHERS (UK)

While women have always helped each other with birth and babies, in many Western cultures, where people are on the move and life is often dominated by the demands of work and career, new mothers can find themselves alone just at the time when they most need company and support. Building a community around a new mother is as important as building a community around the newborn.

Visit from a fairy godmother

"I was totally isolated when I had my first baby," says Katy Smith. "We had moved to a new area when I was eight months pregnant, so I had no time to build a network of friends and my parents were an hour and a half away.

"Dylan was born in hospital and my husband was a dream birth partner; he was just there for me and it was okay for it not to be about him. He is very earthy, practical and calm. But it was a long labour; I was induced and the birth felt out of my control.

I couldn't move. My feet were up in stirrups for an episiotomy, there was blood everywhere. I got the baby out with one last push, and he was fine and beautiful.

"My husband stayed with me until midnight, but after that I remember being awake in a big room, on my own with the baby, trying to feed him but not knowing how to do it. I didn't sleep that night.

"We got home in the cold and ice of November and it was very difficult. I cried and cried and didn't know what to do. My husband was trying his best, but the baby wasn't sleeping and neither was I. I was so wired up I genuinely didn't get any sleep for weeks, so there were just hours and hours to get through with a baby who seemed to be screaming all the time. I was so exhausted and yet I still couldn't sleep.

"The health visitor came regularly as she was worried. One night, I remember banging my head on the wall, trying to hurt myself rather than hurt my baby. No one told me how it can be unbearable when you are so lonely with a new baby.

"My husband tried hard but he didn't understand why I couldn't sleep, even when he took Dylan out of the house for a walk. Once, in the kitchen, he said, 'I miss you.' I said, 'I miss me too.' What I needed was the comfort of female company and to have someone to take care of me.

"Then Sarah, who had been a colleague of mine, came to visit. She was the person who showed me how it should be. She knew me very well and my husband was comfortable with her too. She quietly came one night when Dylan was ten days old. Suddenly, she was there, holding my baby.

"When it's just you alone with the baby it is all: *Need, feed, change nappies, change clothes.* But, when someone else is holding your baby, you can see how beautiful he is.

"So she just held him, changed him, did our washing, fed us, cleared the dishes away. And she said to me, 'You are doing a great job' – even though I knew I wasn't."

> A friend is someone who can find you, even when you can't find yourself.
> – Katy Smith, Yorkshire, UK

"Sarah is now Dylan's godmother. We are both lucky to have her in our lives."

The godmother's tale

Dylan's godmother, Sarah Goldsworthy, says: "When she was seven months pregnant, Katy told me she was moving to Yorkshire – new house, unknown hospital, far from friends and family. I thought she was being very stoical about it, but she reminded me of my younger self; I was twenty-two and very isolated when I had my first child, living in a remote and isolated cottage during a freezing cold winter.

"I remembered that a friend had come to visit me; I had left the new baby to sleep in the next room, but the baby was crying and I was upset, trying to do the right thing. After a while, my friend said, 'Do you think he's going to be a delinquent teenager if you pick him up and feed him now?' So we both laughed, though I was crying and laughing at the same time. That friend made me feel that there was no 'right way' and that I was doing a good job

– and I thought I could be someone like that for Katy.

"When I arrived, I saw a new mum, utterly, utterly exhausted, wanting to do it right and feeling she hadn't a clue. Katy is someone who wants to do everything well, and she was really looking forward to being a mum. I just did the practical things – cooking, cleaning, holding the baby, while all the time saying: 'He's fine, this is normal, you're doing great.'"

> It is like a chain; my friend helped
> me, and I was able to help Katy.
> – Sarah Goldsworthy, Yorkshire, UK

"I know Katy has since done the same for other friends with a new baby. In modern society, it's usually closed doors, keeping people out. There is a sense that you have to do it on your own and if you want support you are weak. We should be helping people find their way, because to be a new mother is one of the most important things you do and yet when it happens you are a complete novice.

"When I was having my own baby, I still remember the voice of the midwife during labour, just her voice, saying, 'Everything is okay, you're doing well.' I was singing a John Denver song, 'Country Road' – although I never got further than the first few lines, which I must have sung hundreds of times. The next day, I heard another woman say, 'Who was singing "Country Road" last night?' I was embarrassed so I didn't reply. Then she said, 'I don't know who it was but I was in the next room, and she really helped me through my delivery.'" ✻ ✻ ✻ ✻

The godfather's witness

Choosing a person to be a godparent to your child is an enormous step – and so is deciding what role a godparent will have in your child's life.

In the Christian tradition, the godparent serves as a sponsor for the child's baptism into the religion, making the Profession of Faith on behalf of an infant. But godparents take on many different roles, depending on the family and its history. In some, a godparent formally accepts responsibility for the child if something should happen to his parents; in others, many godparents may join the family informally, providing the child with a mentor who loves him just as though he is kith and kin.

No matter what your own tradition or choices, the most important step will be talking with the person or people you would like to serve as a godparent about what you *both* want your child to gain from the relationship.

Of course, life will shape their relationship over the years. But the strength of their bond will start in that first conversation, even if your answer is very open-ended, as Bill Savage learned when an old friend and schoolmate asked him to be a godfather to her daughter.

My dear goddaughter, Celine

A few months after you were born in the hallway of your parents' apartment high above Piikoi Street in Honolulu, your mother Dominique, my graduate school-mate, and your father Alan, my childhood friend, invited me to be your godfather. Being a gay man who was not a parent, nor ever thought I would be, and living as I did far away in Thailand, I asked them what was expected of me and whether I was qualified. Your mother's response was, "All you have to do is be there for Celine when she needs you." My reply was, "I can do that."

I am grateful for each of the times we have been together as you have grown into the beautiful, intelligent, deeply open-hearted woman you are. After we knew that Dominique was dying with leukemia, it was a remarkable sight to watch you as a little girl, helping her as she walked on a cane out the door of immigration and customs at the Bangkok airport when your family came to visit. It was not long after that I flew to the Marianas Islands when you were nine years old and your mother had died. That was the first of the times you and I placed flowers in the water for her, and later also for my own late mother and two younger sisters, always returning to the ocean both of us island kids call home. It is one of our practices that I am thankful for.

You have only ever requested me to be there for you once, when you moved to Maui, met someone and asked me to come see that you were alright. I wanted to be with you and him without judgment, to have a different response to your relationship than others had, and I was appreciative of the experience, and in awe at your courage. Your mother may also well have said to me that another expectation was that I would learn as much from her as she would from me, and so I look forward to all else that is still to come.

With much love and respect,

Uncle Bill

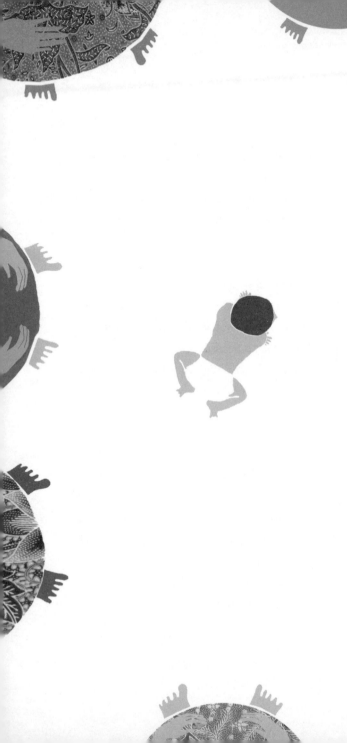

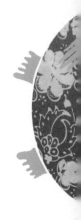

PART 4
THE "FIRST" YEAR

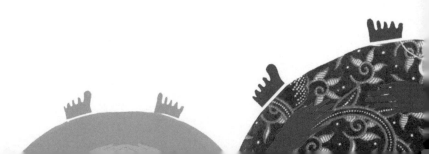

PART 4
THE FIRST YEAR

32

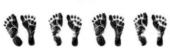

A CUP OF FORTY KEYS:
A YEAR OF "FIRSTS" (PERSIA)

The span of time from conception, through pregnancy and birth is one of profound change in a woman's life. Hard though much of it can be, moving on and letting the child go can be equally daunting. The first year is full of such moments – the first bath, the first haircut, the first steps, the first solid foods. Right up until the first birthday, this is a year when everything is new and special to parent and baby alike.

"In Iran, extended family and communal living are important in the life of a new mother," says Najmieh Batmanglij, the author of *Food of Life: Ancient Persian and Modern Iranian Food and Ceremonies*. "We believe that it takes the whole community to raise a child.

"A new mother needs help and support, not only physically but emotionally, for many weeks after the birth of her child. Our custom is that the mother is pampered by the women of her extended family, usually her mother, sisters and aunts. They cook for her family and take good care of her and the new baby for at least forty days.

"We have special foods too, prepared to restore the strength of the mother, and to nourish her while she is breastfeeding. These are warm, soft, sweet soups and puddings, including *ab gusht-e morgh*, a very rich chicken soup; *shir berenj*, rice pudding; *katchi*, saffron cream; *yakh dar behesht*, also known as 'ice in paradise'; *masqati*, wheat pudding; and a basil seed drink. Our community believes that rice and wheat help to increase the mother's breast milk," Najmieh says.

The first bath

About seven to ten days after the birth, a baby is given the first bath – the *ab e cheleh zadan*. "This is a festive occasion arranged by women friends and family, much like a party for her," explains Najmieh.

"The night before the bath ceremony, one or more close female members of the mother's family will make a paste of egg yolk and chickpea powder, and wrap this around the mother's waist with a cloth."

In some families, a poultice of eggs and lentils was used instead, with honey massaged into the mother's belly. In the morning, she would wear a talisman for good luck. Upon leaving her home for the public bath, mother and baby pass under a Qur'an as a blessing, a melding of old Persian customs with more recent Muslim beliefs.

Many people gather for the ceremony – the midwife, the mother's female friends and family members – and the group sings and claps as they make their way to the bath house. "Then, when she gets to the baths, they massage her whole body for hours with special oils such as nutmeg oil and *roghan-e momyai*; then, they wash her," Najmieh says.

"The women sing together, playing tambourines and *tonbaks* [a traditional Persian drum]. They pass around sweets, fruits and *faludeh*, a rice and saffron ice cream, together with a cold drink made from basil seeds and rosewater syrup."

The meal customarily ended when the new mother ate two boiled eggs and *ghaoot*, a special sweet. The mother's forehead was rubbed with *torbat bibi*, blessed clay – named after the legendary martyr Bibi Shahrbanu, who some say is associated with Anahita, the Persian "goddess of waters".

"Forty days after the birth, the women repeat the same ceremony at the baths, but this time they concentrate on the baby in order to welcome and purify it," says Najmieh. A specially engraved brass or copper *jam e chehel klid* ("cup of forty keys") is filled with water and blessed, and then the mother holds the baby above her head as water from the cup is poured on the infant.

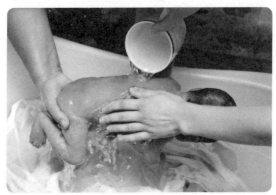

Baby's first bath

Nush-e jan! ("Food of life")

Najmieh Batmanglij (najmiehskitchen.com) offers these recipes from her book *Food of Life: Ancient Persian and Modern Iranian Food and Ceremonies*, which was published in a special twenty-fifth anniversary edition in 2011.

Shir Berenj (Rice Pudding)

Ingredients

½ cups rice, washed
2 cups water
¼ tsp sea salt
3 cups milk or almond milk
½ cup cream
¼ cup rose water
1 tsp ground cardamom
½ cup grape molasses or honey
1 cup pomegranate arils (in season)
½ cup ground raw pistachios

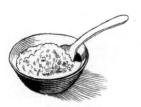

Method

Place the rice in a medium saucepan with 2 cups water and the salt. Bring to a boil and reduce to a medium heat. Cover and cook for 20 minutes, or until the rice is tender. Add the milk and cream and return to a boil. Reduce to a low heat, cover and cook for 55 minutes, stirring occasionally. Add rose water and cardamom, and cook over low heat for 15 to 20 minutes longer, or until the mixture has thickened to a pudding consistency. Remove from the heat, spoon into serving bowls and chill. Top with grape molasses, pistachio and pomegranate. Serves 6.

Katchi (Saffron Cream)

Ingredients
5½ cups water
2½ cups sugar
1 tsp ground saffron dissolved in ¼ cup hot water
¼ cup rose water
½ tsp ground cardamom
1 cup unsalted butter or vegetable oil
2 cups all-purpose flour
2 tbsp slivered almonds
2 tbsp slivered pistachios

Method
Bring the water and sugar to a boil in a saucepan. Add the saffron water, rose water and cardamom. Remove syrup from heat and set aside to cool. Melt the butter in a deep skillet, gradually adding the flour while stirring constantly with a wooden spoon. Cook the roux over medium heat for about 20 to 25 minutes, or until it is golden brown. Add the saffron syrup to the roux, stirring quickly and constantly. Simmer until the mixture gains a creamy consistency. Add warm water if it becomes too thick. Transfer to a bowl and garnish with nuts. Serve warm. Serves 6.

Sharbat-e gol-e Mhammadi (Rose Water Syrup with Basil Seeds)

Ingredients
2½ cups water
4 cups sugar
¼ cup fresh lime juice
½ cup rose water
1 cup basic seeds (*tokhm-e sharbati*), soaked in 2 cups water for 3 to 4 hours

Method
In a laminated pot, bring the water and sugar to a boil, then simmer for 10 minutes. Add the lime juice, rose water and basil seed mixture, and cook for a further 10 minutes. Remove pot from heat and allow to cool. In a pitcher, mix 1 part syrup, 3 parts water and 2 ice cubes per person. Stir and serve well chilled. Yields 1 pint.

The means of grace

The year before I gave birth to our daughter, I took my husband, Dan, to visit my extended family in Friesland, the Netherlands, for the first time. One of the places I showed him was the church my family has attended for centuries, and the cemetery surrounding it that contains the graves of my ancestors. Frisian names are nothing if not unique – my husband couldn't begin to pronounce most of the words on the headstones, Geertje and Eelkje and Baukje to name just a few – but they sound like home to me. So, when I became pregnant later that year, it wasn't hard to choose a meaningful name, one shared by a great-grandmother, a special aunt and my sister (and one that's a little easier to pronounce than most Frisian names): Hendrica.

Our Hendrica was born three months early following a traumatic delivery that nearly ended my life. Weighing only two and a half pounds, she was immediately whisked away to the NICU, and it was there that Dan saw our fragile baby – hooked up to a ventilator, feeding tube and monitors for her heart, lungs, blood pressure and oxygen level – for the first time. He stood by her Plexiglas box weeping, he later told me, and a kind nurse told him that he didn't have to cry. Our baby would be in the hospital for a few months, the nurse said, but she would grow.

"Should we have her baptized now?" Dan asked.

✳ ✳

It was his way of asking if things would *really* be okay in the end. Was our daughter at risk of dying soon? And, when the nurse said no, we didn't need to do that, she was telling him that Hendrica would live.

In Isaiah 43, the Lord says, "Do not fear, for I have redeemed you; I have called you by name, you are mine." And God knew Hendrica's name then, before her baptism, just as God knows and loves the names of children from all sorts of faiths and backgrounds. But the truth is we felt nothing *but* fear after Hendrica's birth. We were heartsick that we couldn't even hold our little one for several weeks. And so we prayed, sending our hopes upward, an act that is, for me, as mysterious as it is helpful.

Others prayed too, members of our scrappy urban Lutheran church among them, who also brought meals and transportation and love to our home when the bassinet stood empty by our bed. And then the happy day came when they stood up with us, faced the baptismal font and prayed when Hendrica was finally baptized, wearing a long, beautiful one-hundred-year-old gown that had been worn by her father and grandmother before her.

Baptism is a sacrament, a Christian ceremony that reminds us that we are born into a fallen and flawed world, but with the waters of baptism are reborn as children of God. It's sometimes also called a christening, or a naming ceremony. And, just as

Hendrica's first and last names connect her to the history of both her parents, her baptism was a way to connect her to the larger family of faith into which she was born.

But it was the present community that we most wanted to acknowledge. Here was our family: my brother and Dan's sister standing by our sides, happy in their new roles as godparents. Here was our church family, celebrating this new life. And across the globe was the larger family of Christian faith that has been a great source of hope for her parents.

Hendrica was finally home.

– Helen Atsma, New York, USA

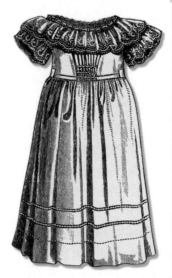

Victorian christening gown

33

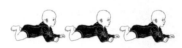

BABY'S WEIGHT IN GOLD:
AQIQAH (ISLAM)

The formal naming ceremony, *'aqiq* (قيق), traditionally takes place seven days after the baby's birth, and is one of the *sunnah* of Islam – a highly recommended practice. It is a ceremony of thanksgiving. The baby's hair is shaved and a sacrifice (*aqiqah*, "to cut") is made – according to Hadith 2829 of Abu Dawud.

Sarah Javaid, who works for MADE (Muslim Agency for Development Education) in Europe, remembers the many rituals of her son's *aqiqah*. "Some people have a big party with lots of people, but, as I was still feeling a little sore after the birth, we decided that we'd keep it small and informal with immediate family.

"We shaved baby Kamran's head and then weighed his hair on the scales. The tradition is to give the equivalent amount in money to charity [called *sadaqah* in Arabic]. With my English genes, Kamran was born with very little hair – it weighed in at zero grams on the scales! We made a donation anyway, as it is customary to do so and brings blessing for the baby and the family."

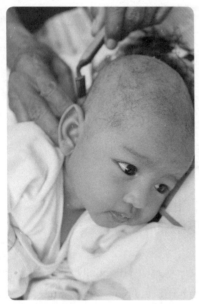

Shaving baby's hair as part of an *aqiqah*, Malaysia

Traditionally, the donation is made in gold or silver of equal weight to the hair.

Sarah goes on: "The other *aqiqah* custom is for a sheep to be slaughtered – two for a boy and one for a girl – and for the meat to be distributed to poor people who would not often get the opportunity to eat meat." The idea, interpreted from the Hadith, is that this will ensure a sweet disposition in the child. Often the right back leg of the animal is given to the midwife, since Fatimah, a daughter of the Prophet Muhammad, is said to have done so.

"Many Muslims who live in the UK arrange for this distribution of meat to be done in another country, and we did ours in Bangladesh," says Sarah. "But some also do it in the UK, and you often find a tired-looking dad at the door with a big bag of meat a few days after a baby has been born!

"It's a really nice way for the wider community to share in the celebration of the baby's birth."

34

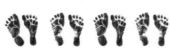

FIRST DATE NIGHT:
RECONNECTING AT HOME

How soon is it safe, or wise, or even pleasurable to have sex after childbirth?

Ibu Srihartati Pandi, of White Ribbon Alliance Indonesia, says the answer is clear: "In our country, we believe that men should not sleep with their wives for forty days after the birth of a baby. This is for the good of the mother's health."

In Uganda, according to Samuel Senfuka, "No sex is allowed during the postnatal period; her husband's conjugal rights are suspended during this time. She is in confinement so that her husband is not tempted. This lasts until the umbilical cord is dry. She sleeps in the living room, apart from her husband so that he cannot pressurize or force her into sex. This is a good way to preserve her health."

The forty-day rule is common in many cultures. It's no coincidence that this is the amount of time it can take for the uterus to return to normal and for the flow of lochia to slowly diminish and come to an end. (*Lochia* comes from the Greek word meaning "relating to childbirth" and refers to the vaginal discharge that all mothers experience after birth.)

Whether your thoughts about when to start having sex again are based on health considerations, or influenced by traditional or cultural expectations, above all this is – or should be – a woman's personal decision.

Making time for two

Of all the life events that can ambush your sex life, one of the most significant is having a baby. It may get better, it may get worse, but chances are it will never be quite the same again.

On the plus side, pregnancy can be a time of tremendous sensuality and heightened pleasure, while having a baby is a profound experience, which can leave women feeling strong, attractive and confident as never before. Consider the stories of some recent mothers, who asked not to be named.

> We carried on having sex right up until the time of the birth. In fact, the baby was overdue and we had been told that sex can trigger labour. But I had no idea what to expect after the birth. I had a small tear and some stitches; to my surprise, breastfeeding made me feel very sexual. We lay together one night and ended up having sex; he said, "the last person here was our baby" – just acknowledging that made it alright.

Women who have had difficult births may be left with a sense of trauma. But, even when the birth has been a good one, broken nights, breastfeeding and postnatal bleeding can add up to a period of celibacy. Sex is on hold for months. Nature also wants us to finish (fully) breastfeeding one baby before we start another, and so breastfeeding women produce exceptionally high levels of prolactin, a hormone that can suppress a woman's libido.

> I've done all the holding all day long. By the time I get into bed at night, I just want to be held myself...

And then there is the mysterious phenomenon of "baby's intuition":

> How is it that babies always seem to know when you are – at last – starting to resume your sex life? Is it because they don't want you to make a rival baby, or are they just natural killjoys? It never failed to happen. For the first year of our baby's life, he would wake up just at the crucial moment; not in the early stages when you wouldn't mind too much, but just at the point where you are left incredibly frustrated!

Thankfully, this doesn't last forever:

> Now that I am starting to sleep through the night again, my libido is gradually coming back. Sex gets better later on when you've reached a level of ease with each other. Your husband has been with you or supported you in giving birth and becoming a mother; he loves and respects you – the real you – and you love him back. That is a wonderful time.

Getting down to business

Whether or not you think you're ready to restart your sex life, follow these tips:

* Wait until you genuinely feel ready, and forget about the six-week check-up, which in some countries is the date at which any stitches from delivery are considered healed – that's not some official time at which resuming sex is recommended.

* If you notice any deep sighs or huffs from the other side of the bed, talk it over; communication is essential. But choose your time carefully: in the middle of the night when the baby is crying is not the time to raise the subject.

* Experiment and find new and various ways to give each other pleasure. Start slowly and sensuously; don't rush it.

* The hormones produced while breastfeeding can also interfere with vaginal lubrication, causing uncomfortable dryness. So, again, take it slowly and sensuously, and try experimenting with a lubricant.

And here are some tips for the person on the other side of the bed too:

* Take the new mother in your life out somewhere pleasant and relaxing, and set aside any hopes for

a steamy evening. Instead, catch up on each other's feelings, and then raise the topic gently: "I am
really missing making love to you. How do you feel
about it?" Accept the reply she gives you, even if it
is: "I just don't feel like it at the moment."

❖ Ask her if there is something she would enjoy in
the meantime, like a massage, and when you get
home, try it…

❖ Don't wait until the baby has finally dropped off to
sleep at one in the morning to suggest sex – that's
the time to grab some much-needed rest.

❖ Don't prod her in the back or make a grab at her,
roll over in a huff or bleat her name in a desperate
voice – that will mostly serve to alarm her, annoy
her or up her anxiety levels, which may be much
higher than you realize.

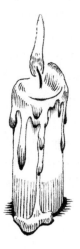

✗ ✗ ✗ ✗ ✗ ✗ ✗ ✗ ✗ ✗ ✗ ✗ ✗ ✗ ✗

Egg heads

In Moldovan tradition, when a
woman wants to stop breastfeeding, she places many
eggs in the room where the
baby sleeps. If the child pays
attention to the eggs and
points to any of them, then
he is ready to be weaned.

35

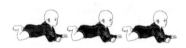

LETTING GO:
FIRST TASTE OF *PASNI* (NEPAL)

In the Hindu communities of Nepal, when a baby girl is five months old or a baby boy is six months, a *pasni*, or weaning ceremony, is held. At this celebration, babies are fed their first solid food – rice.

First, an auspicious date and time is chosen by an astrologer, and all the closest relatives are invited to take part. The customs around the day vary according to religion, caste and location, explains Samjhana Phuyal of Nepal. "For instance, Brahmins serve *kheer* to the baby, which is a rice pudding cooked with milk and sugar, but a myriad of different rice dishes are prepared and served in Newar [the traditional name for the Kathmandu Valley]. Traditionally, all these rice dishes were served on one giant woven plate of leaves. But today people will serve the rice dish in a silver bowl with a gold spoon."

✖ ✖ ✖ ✖

Sacred saffron

Samjhana remembers the rituals of the day: "Our baby was dressed for the occasion in saffron-coloured silk clothes. My mother held her while the entire family took turns to feed her the first taste of rice. After she had eaten, there was another extensive *puja* led by the priest and accompanied by chanting from ancient scriptures. Sometimes the oldest member of the household or clan will perform these chants instead.

"For the rest of the day, our baby wore a special outfit made of red velvet and embroidered with silver and golden thread. Though she wore the outfit all day, it is believed that the child should not wear the outfit again after this ceremony. My baby

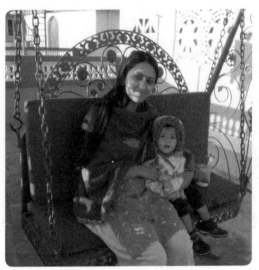

Samjhana and her daughter

daughter was offered gifts and money by close relatives, and gold and silver ornaments by her grandparents and others. These ornaments include heavy silver *kalli* (anklets) carved with a dragon at both ends to keep bad spirits away from the baby. These ornaments are often handed down the generations, as heirlooms."

Samjhana says that in recent years *pasni* ceremonies have become extremely lavish in Nepal. "Large parties are held not just for close relatives, but also for colleagues and friends. The guests, numbering in their hundreds, partake in a wedding-style banquet under tents, which are often catered by companies," she explains. "The guests also now bring gifts for the child, a new custom that has become more popular with the commercial rise of clothes, toys and other gift items targeted towards children. However, simpler ceremonies are still performed in temples dedicated to female Tantric deities, with only a few relatives in attendance."

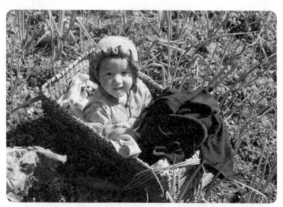

Baby in basket cot, Nepal

Served with a side of rock

Okuizome (食初), literally "first eat", is the Japanese cele-bration of the baby's weaning, traditionally held when the baby is one hundred days old (even though the baby is most likely still breastfeeding). The paternal grandmother prepares a family feast, and each adult is served a small pebble – everyone bites down on the pebble to wish the baby a life with strong teeth – and no hunger.

The meal traditionally includes fish, vegetables, a clear broth, *umeboshi* (pickled plum) and *sekihan* (a ceremonial sticky red rice), and the parents will press each of the foods against the baby's lips, to mimic eating it.

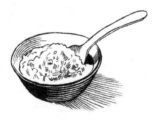

36

MAMA, BABA, NANA, PAPA: FIRST WORDS

How has it come about that the first words for "mother" and "father" are so similar in so many countries?

In the 1950s, American anthropologist George P. Murdoch examined these words in 470 languages and found that "mother" had the sound *ma*, *me* or *mo* in fifty-two percent of the languages in his sample, while "father" had *pa* or *po*, or *ta* or *to*, in fifty-five percent of them.

How could this be? Perhaps because the easiest sounds to utter are those made entirely with the lips, sounds like *em*, *buh* and *puh* – and so they are the first consonants produced by babies. Of these, *em* is slightly easier to make; the *buh* and *puh* sounds require a bit more work at the back of the mouth. And so the very first sounds produced by babies are usually of the form *mama*, swiftly followed by *baba* and *papa*.

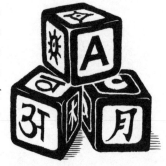

Of course, what happens next is that parents respond with delight to the sound, assuming that our babies are trying to speak to us – when, in fact, they are just babbling! We then speak back to our babies, owning that first word. And thus baby talk enters adult languages all over the world.

Language	mother sound	father sound
Apalai (Amazon)	aya	papa
Basque (Spain)	ama	aita
Chechen (Russia)	naana	daa
Cree (Canada)	mama	papa
Dakota (USA)	ena	ate
English	mama, mummy, mommy	papa, dada, daddy
French	maman	papa
Georgian	deda	mama
Hungarian	anya	apa
Kikuyu (East Africa)	nana	baba
Kobon (New Guinea)	amy	bap
Korean	eomma, eomeoni	appa, abeoji
Luo (Kenya)	mama	baba
Malay	emak	bapa
Mandarin (China)	mama, muqin	baba, fuqin
Nahuatl (Mexico)	naan	ta'
Pipil (El Salvador)	naan	tatah
Quechua (Ecuador)	mama	tayta
Romanian	mama	tata
Russian	mama	papa, tata, tyatya
Spanish	mamá, mami	papá, dádi

Swahili (East Africa)	mama	baba
Tagalog (Philippines)	nánay, ináy	tátay
Tamil (Sri Lanka)	amma, thaii	appa, thanthai
Tibetan	amma	ppa
Turkish	ana, anne	baba
Urdu (India)	mang	bap
Welsh	mam	tad
Xhosa (South Africa)	mama	tata

Listen and explain

In the first few months of your new baby's life, everything is guesswork.

They cry, and you try to work out why.

They sleep and you wonder how long for.

They feed and you marvel at what has made them so hungry.

But, from the moment they begin to speak and understand language, there are two words that you'll need to drum into yourself: "listen" and "explain".

Fail to listen, and you won't understand their problem; fail to explain and they won't understand yours. It may take more patience than you're willing or able to give, but it's the single most important thing I've learned about parenting: listen and explain.

Oh, and hug. That's the fun part.

– Rebecca Front, BAFTA award-winning actor on The Thick of It and Inspector Morse, UK

We *are* family

For us, it was impossible not to tell everyone I was pregnant with our first child the minute the two blue lines showed up on the stick. As a lesbian couple, my partner, Rowena, and I had been working on starting our family for eight years. As it is for many other broody lesbians, it was a rocky, emotional journey through the methods available to us: looking at adoption, asking male friends to donate sperm, getting to know a gay couple who might want to co-parent, going to a clinic for insemination, meeting sperm donors through the Web. We shared the ups and commiserated over the downs, turning to our family and friends for support when we needed it.

We were such open books that it was the first thing people asked about whenever they saw us. So, aside from our initial disbelief that home insemination had worked on the first attempt after such a long journey (and after four failed clinic inseminations), we couldn't contain ourselves.

We told my mum first, as she was battling cancer and needed something positive to focus on – her first grandchild seemed perfect. She burst into tears of joy and between chemo treatments she threw herself into enjoying my pregnancy, making baby clothes and buying gifts like any other excited grandmother-to-be. All our families and friends were overjoyed and probably a bit relieved to not have to listen to us go on about wanting children any more! Noah was born in August 2010.

The second time around, we managed to keep a lid on it until the first scan. Just like many other middle-class couples in their late thirties, we preferred to err on the side of caution and wait until we were in the safer zone of established pregnancy with a lower risk of miscarriage before sharing the news. It felt odd to lie to people, because, of course, they had started to ask again – by then, Noah was two. We'd been trying for a year so we found various ways to distract or throw people off the scent. Eli arrived in March 2013.

There are other things people always ask. If they are feeling brave, they will go straight for the jugular – the donor father. *What is his role? What are you going to tell your children? What will they call him?* With my second pregnancy, the first question usually was: *Is it the same father?* We've never minded people's curiosity, as we are very open and happy to educate the world on lesbian parenting. But it does expose us to lots of quite invasive questions.

Another area of interest is names. *What surname will you give your children? What will they call you?* Lesbian mums-to-be spend a lot of time on these decisions. The surname issue is common among many couples in the modern world, where women no longer always take a husband's name, but the issue of how to have your child differentiate between two mummies is not. Some mums go for "Mummy Lisa" and "Mummy Karen", some go for "Mummy" and "Mumma", or a variant nickname, or simply first names. At the end of the day, the child takes the lead. I've been called "Mummy",

"Mum", "Hannah", "Anna", even Rowena's usual moniker, "Mumma", depending on whether Noah is making a joke, asserting his independence or experimenting. Rowena wanted him to stick to "Mummena" for her, but he defaults back to "Mumma".

We deliberate over these things, trying to make our family unit as "normal" as possible to minimize any possibility that our differences affect our children in any negative way. We just want to be accepted as parents, as a family.

As gay rights catch up and same-sex parents become more visible, our difference is becoming less of an issue, but our societal rules aren't there yet. We may have civil partnerships and both be on our sons' birth certificates, but we can still feel invisible.

Not long ago, we went to a lesbian festival in the Midlands. Rowena popped out to the local supermarket with our son, Noah, to get supplies. There were quite a few women from the festival in there, but when Rowena got to the till the man serving her lowered his voice and confided, "I've served *so* many lesbians today, I don't know why!" To him, a woman with a child was automatically heterosexual.

Such invisibility is felt acutely by LGBT parents. It's partly what led me to start *We Are Family* magazine (www.wearefamilymagazine.co.uk), celebrating, supporting and normalizing LGBT families here. It has been the biggest, most passionate thing I have done to celebrate my unique family.

— *Hannah Latham, Bristol, UK*

37

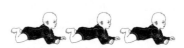

FIRST STEPS:
TEDAK SITEN (INDONESIA)

"*Tedak siten* is our traditional Javanese feast for when a couple's first baby first walks, at about seven months old," says Dr Srihartati Pandi of White Ribbon Alliance Indonesia, in collaboration with Stikes Mitra Ria Husada, who have trained more than six hundred midwives in the past decade. "We celebrate the first time that the sole of the baby's foot touches the ground."

It is an elaborate ceremony meant to prepare the child for life, and like such ceremonies around the world it has many layers of meaning. Most essentially, it marks the moment when the child first connects with the Earth.

The ceremony begins with the mother and father bowing their heads to the grandparents. The parents ask for blessings and pray for the gods to protect their child.

Then, says Ibu Pandi, "the parents will hold and guide their child while she steps on seven cakes of *jadah*, or sticky rice, which is made in seven colours including white, red, blue, yellow, purple, black and orange. These colours represent the different challenges

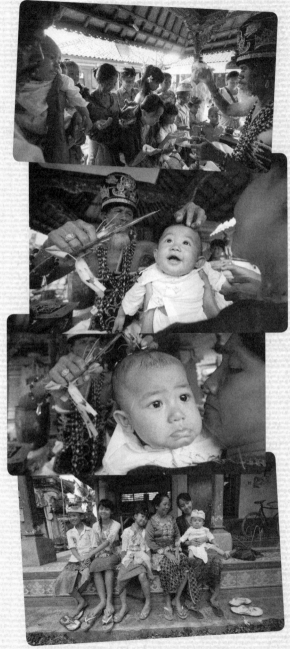

In Javanese *tedak* means "to step" and
siti means "earth"

the child will face on the path of life, and how she will overcome them, while the number seven is symbolic of the seven layers of heaven."

The parents help the child to climb a series of steps made from sticks of sugar cane. This expresses the parents' hope that the child will have strength and perseverance through life, according to Ibu Pandi. Then the child is seated in a bamboo cage – of the kind used to keep chickens, she explains. "The cage symbolizes how the child is cared for by the parents, but also shows that he or she will belong to society and accept its laws."

She continues: "In the cage are little objects – such as a ball, a car, money, writing implements, a book, jewellery, a musical instrument. The family watches to see which object the child will pick up – as this symbolizes the future profession that may be chosen by the child. If a baby chooses a book, it means that he or she may be a teacher; if a kitchen utensil, the child could be a cook or housewife, and so on.

"Next the child is bathed in a brass basin with flowers of seven colours including jasmine and rose petals, showing how the child will bring good fragrance. Then the parents will cut into a special rice dish, *tumpeng*, while asking for God's blessings.

"Finally, the parents throw *empon empon*, a yellow rice mixed with coins, to their guests, demonstrating generosity to their community."

In sharing this custom, Ibu Pandi spoke with Dina Sintadewi Landini of White Ribbon Alliance.

✳ ✳ ✳ ✳

Walking out into the world

In a child's first year, mother and baby are still so deeply connected that every change and every new development is greeted with delight – but also with a certain pang. A mother knows that her child is beginning the long process of leaving babyhood and growing up. Even when she understands how right and good this is, she may also feel that a precious time is coming to an end. Soon enough, the toddler will be an adult, ready to leave the home and walk the world on his own. Until then, there are ways to ease the transitions.

* The walking cure: When a baby begins to crawl in Bhutan, she is massaged with mustard oil and placed in the sun to increase her strength.

* The long walk ahead: Among the Quechua of the Andes, until a baby starts to walk, both sexes are dressed in girls' clothing and their hair is left long. Around the time of the child's first steps, a ritual hair-cutting ceremony is held, during which he is publicly named and identified by gender. The

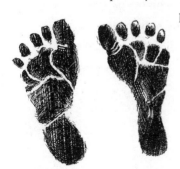

parents bestow the child with a first inheritance – usually a baby animal or some rows of plants in one of their fields – as a first step into life.

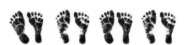

38

EL SALTO DEL COLACHO: PROTECT THIS BABY (SPAIN)

Any new parent knows that sense of passionate love for the new baby, which is coupled with horror at the idea of anything going terribly wrong. Even those who do not believe in God will still say "God forbid" that anything bad should happen. At the mildest threat, we may "cross our fingers" in hopes that this will ensure all will be well, thus invoking the power of the Christian cross to keep our loved ones safe.

In our modern world of antibiotics and paediatric visits, there is a safety net against infection and disease for those who are able to get health care, but for most of human history parents have felt that they are at the mercy of mysterious, sometimes fickle, forces that they could not control. And they did all they could to ward off evil.

Do not answer!

After the baby is born, the mother stays in a separate room, and the father and others come and see the baby. We stay indoors in this room for a week, and only go out to use the toilet.

Very few people must come in when you are resting for the first week. If someone even calls your name, you should not reply, as it might be a bad person who will harm you and the baby.

– *Afande Jephrace and Esther Sikote, Luiya people, Kenya, in conversation with the Belaku Trust*

Devil's play

The spectacle of *El Salto del Colacho*, meaning "The Devil's Jump", is held every spring as part of the Catholic Feast of Corpus Christi in the village of Castrillo de Murcia in northern Spain.

The Corpus Christi festival's annual procession of flag bearers, drummers, dancers and bell ringers also includes some men dressed in red and yellow costumes, which are meant to make them look like the Devil, *El Colacho*. On the final Sunday of the feast, a series of mattresses are laid around the procession route. Babies, sometimes six at a time, are laid on a mattress, awaiting *El Colacho*, who will cavort around and then leap over them.

El Salto del Colacho reflects the desire to cleanse the newborn of original sin. As the jumper passed over the baby, any evil would be attracted to this personification of evil, and would follow him, leaving the baby's soul cleansed.

This notorious display dates back to 1620 or 1621, and takes place sixty days after Easter. In recent years, the Vatican has noted that baby jumping is potentially dangerous, and should not be considered part of religious observance.

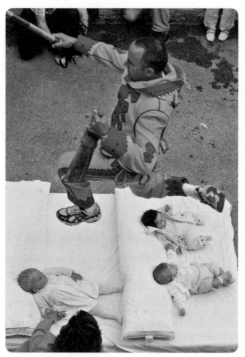

El Colacho jumping over infants

✖ ✖ ✖ ✖

A loan from the spirits

We believe that, like the elders of our community, babies are very close to the spirit world. If you don't treat them well, they will be taken back by the spirits. That is why we say never go to a funeral when pregnant, or to a wake. We also say to always speak well of others when you are pregnant because it will come back upon the baby if you don't. And we never buy anything for the baby until it is born or it is bad luck.

This is because children are on loan to us. We don't own them, they are not ours.

– *Julie Lys, Métis nurse, Northwest Territories, Canada*

Tempting evil in other ways

Midwife Sharlene Daly recalls two Albanian traditions for warding off the "evil eye". She says breastfeeding was to be kept hidden, since mother and baby are both vulnerable during this time. In addition, "a patch of garlic would be placed under the baby's pillow in the pram, or under the clothes on the chest, to protect her".

That seems much less dangerous than baby jumping, but it's also true that the parents who put their babies in the way of *El Colacho* clearly care very much for the safety of them. And the Spanish ritual is not the only one in which parents have tempted fate in order to ensure a baby is safe.

Take a similarly risky-looking tradition of baby throwing at the Baba Umer *dargah*, an ancient shrine, in the village of Musti, India, about three hundred miles south of Mumbai. Parents – both Hindu and Muslim – ask to have their children dangled from the shrine and then dropped onto a blanket held trampoline-style below them. Like *El Salto del Colacho*, this is not a common event, and the tradition has been widely condemned by religious and community leaders alike. So why would any parent risk it?

The answer is that the parents believe that going through the ritual will be good for their babies, drawing evil out of or away from them and bringing prosperity – rather as Christians believe that baptism in holy water will help to nullify the stain of "original sin". As with a baptism, if a baby is upset it is only a matter of seconds before she is back in the arms of her loving parents.

But it goes without saying – please don't try any of these feats at home!

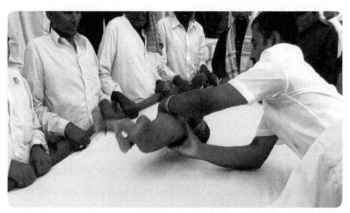

At the Baba Umer *dargah* (shrine), India

The Serbian rattle of good fortune

The father, with his mother-in-law, must prepare the house for the baby's arrival, buying all the necessities for the baby. It is considered to be bad luck to buy anything or start any preparation before the baby arrives.

When the mother and baby arrive home, they are not supposed to go out for forty days. Mothers are supposed to rest and spend time with the baby. During this period, close family and friends visit and help out. When a grandmother visits the mother and baby for the first time, it is called *babine* (*baba* means "grandmother"). The grandmother brings certain foods – roast chicken, homemade bread and cake – and everyone sits together and eats the feast.

Guests usually bring a present for the baby, but the closest family, particularly grandparents and godparents, give money too – they leave the money under the baby's pillow. If the first baby is a boy, they often give an engraved golden coin – a *dukat*. The rattling of coins for the baby symbolizes not just wealth, but also happiness.

People also used to lace up a red ribbon around the baby's wrist to fight the *protiv uroka* ("evil spirits"). The ribbon stays on the baby's wrist until baptism, which should happen within the baby's first year.

– *Jelena Vulinovic-Zlatan, London, UK*

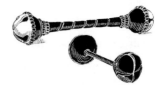

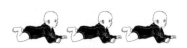

39

A NUDGE INTO THE FUTURE:
DOLJABI (KOREA)

D *ol* is the celebration of a child's first one hundred days of life – the first birthday – in Korea. For it, a special *tol*, or table, is prepared. A dozen or more varieties of *ddeok* (rice cakes) are laid out, often stacked to show off their colours in layers, along with a bowl of rice and other delicacies – pineapple, oranges and other fruit, and candies and cakes are often set out. The baby is dressed in a special *dol-bok* outfit, complemented with a *dol-ddi* (a long belt that symbolizes longevity) and a *dol-jumuni* (a pouch that symbolizes the luck to be carried through life).

This birthday feast and custom is a prelude to the main event: *doljabi* (돌잔치), a kind of fortune-telling exercise intended to show what the child will become in his future life. The child is presented with a low table full of objects, all within his reach. Whatever the child chooses to grasp is seen as representing what he will go on to do in his life. For instance, a stack of coins or bills, or a bowl of rice, means the child will be wealthy or have a life of plenty; a long piece of string or a spool of thread means

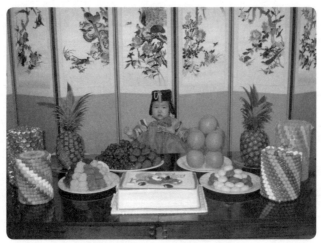

Baby posed for *doljabi* portrait

he will have a long life; a pencil or book means a life filled with scholarship. Today, families often place non-traditional items on the table to represent possible career paths: a stethoscope (becoming a doctor or carer), a microphone or TV remote control (a career in entertainment), a computer mouse (a job in high tech) or sporting equipment (athletic prowess).

Divine future

There is something literally divine about babies. Who are they? Where have they come from? Why?

As Stephen, the partner and guru of legendary midwife Ina May Gaskin, puts it in Gaskin's book *Spiritual Midwifery*, "when a child is born the entire Universe has to shift and make room...A newborn infant is just as intelligent as you are, [but] just doesn't speak your language yet."

Dream with a smile

What do I want for my daughter? Oxbridge...Badminton... Klosters...But seriously, in the current climate I would settle for a kind husband who doesn't want too many camels. I could probably find llamas; they're quite prolific round these parts.
– *Hamish Guerrini, the White Rabbit from Glastonbury Festival's Rabbit Hole and Mad Cows frontman*

The Romantic poet William Wordsworth expressed similar sentiments in 'Intimations of Mortality':

> Our birth is but a sleep and a forgetting:
> The soul that rises with us, our life's star,
> Hath had elsewhere its setting,
> And cometh from afar.
> Not in entire forgetfulness,
> And not in utter nakedness,
> But trailing clouds of glory, do we come
> From God, who is our home:
> Heaven lies about us in our infancy.

Many rituals honour this perception of the spiritual in the newborn, and the belief that a baby's future is in the hands of the divine:

❖ Never leave things *just* to fate: "In Nepal there is a merry celebration once the baby has made it to the sixth day of life," says Samjhana Phuyal. "On this day, the infant is bathed, adorned with new clothes and massaged with oil in order to please the gods of fate. Then, as the child sleeps, a *peepul* leaf plate containing raw rice is placed on the headrest or shelf above the baby's cot. An oil lamp is lit, and placed on the shelf together with a blank sheet of paper and a new pen. This is done as a ritual to please the gods, who will come to write down the fate of the child. The rice is given to make sure the gods are well disposed towards the baby."

❖ Acknowledge your teething troubles: The Armenian *agra hadig* takes place around the time that a child's first tooth comes in. Symbolic items are placed before the child, and then a piece of lace is placed on the baby's head and barley pearls are poured over it. The first item the baby picks up after that symbolizes her future.

❖ Embrace your fruitful dreams: In Tibet, when the mother has auspicious dreams it means her child is going to have a good life. Good fortune can be seen if the dreamer is picking and eating fruit, comes across a white conch shell or jewellery, hears music playing or witnesses the sun rising. Bad dreams – such as dreams of darkness, of falling or being lost, having arguments, or of weeping and drowning – suggest the child is not destined to see much luck.

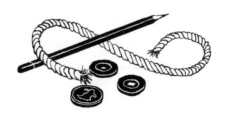

A mother's gift

The majestic gift of becoming a mother cannot be written in words. It is the most unique and supreme position that life can give you, and I have cherished every single precious moment.

I do believe that, through all of life's obstacles and adventures, to be a mother is the finest thing I have ever done.

Gazing into my new little girls' eyes gave both Andrew and I the golden cord that comes from becoming parents, and, for me, a mother.

My girls and I are united and we call ourselves "the tripod". It is the best role I have and I cherish the joy of guiding two bright shining souls. I have never controlled them, I realize they are their own beings, I simply remain consistent and steadfast to truth. I believe, if you speak total truth to your children, they grow to trust you, and that trust brings respect and unconditional love.

There are different ways of mothering, but I have always maintained a constant force of spiritual strength as well as humility and manners. I always say, "Nobody wants to see a grumpy Princess. If you are not going to smile, then don't go out!"

I remember, when my girls came home from school, I would shut the door, turn my telephone off, turn the television off and just sit still and wait for them to talk. Sometimes the best mothering comes from being silent and listening.

One key point is that I never forget I was a child and I had fears and worries, and just because I am now a mother, does it mean you put away your "own child"? I think not!

Every single day I have spent in this world, I have pushed against the boundary fences of life. When writing this, I realize how special it is to be able to just say it as it is. To truly create, or to write creatively, is to choose a subject close to your heart, and have no doubts about your feelings. So then, write them down. For me, nothing is better than writing about my darling girls and the enormity of the love that fills my heart and makes my life complete.

– Sarah Ferguson, Duchess of York

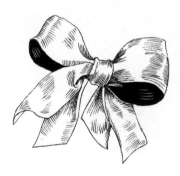

Step into your power

The broad idea of mothering is something that I truly honour. It has not only fuelled my ability to give birth to my daughters, but to give birth to my business, my foundation, my passions. It informs the respect I have for life in every state, past, present and future, and it bolsters my dream for the daughters of the world to preserve culture, empower children and propel integrative health forward so that every woman has the opportunity to step into her own power.

– Donna Karan, fashion designer, founder of the Urban Zen Foundation and White Ribbon Alliance Champion, USA

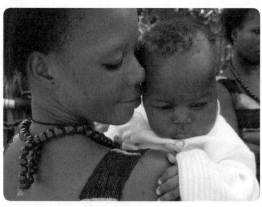

Mother and baby, Burkina Faso

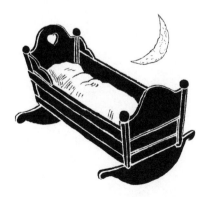

40

FINAL WISDOM:
COMING FULL CIRCLE

So there we have it. Threads of wisdom woven by the hands of women since the human race began. Dropped in times of crisis and conflict; picked up again and reconnected in times and places of peace and prosperity.

The same customs of opening doors and windows, untying knots and necklaces, happen at births divided by continents among peoples who have never crossed paths. Traditions of celebrating pregnancy, supporting birth, welcoming and naming children are richly various but universal. Taboo behaviours, practices and attitudes guide us at a deep level, across divides of culture and religion. Special items of clothing for pregnancy and birth, delicious and nutritious recipes and herbs, heartfelt prayers and poems in many languages echo each other around the world.

All tapping into the same sense that, while birth is basically the same powerfully physical process for all women everywhere, it is also a profound mystery. Becoming a mother bonds our mind, body and spirit, connecting us to our ancestors in a tapestry of wisdom that reaches far back into the past, even as we create the future.

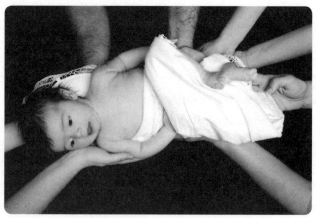

Infant held by many hands

ABOUT

WHITE RIBBON ALLIANCE

If we can fix things for mothers – and we can – we can fix so many other things that are wrong in the world. Women are at the heart of every family, every nation. You just can't build healthy peaceful, prosperous societies without making life better for women and girls.

– *Sarah Brown, Global Patron of White Ribbon Alliance*

It remains a scandal that childbirth is the biggest killer of young women in many countries; eight hundred mothers still die every day, and almost all of these deaths are preventable.

Over a decade ago, White Ribbon Alliance formed because the voices of women at risk of dying in childbirth were not being heard. We rapidly grew as thousands of people and groups joined the network, speaking as one voice, identifying problems in their own communities and finding specific solutions at a national level across Africa and Asia. We are now the leading coalition of advocates for maternal health, uniting citizens to demand the right to a safe birth for every woman, everywhere.

We have made progress; deaths are down by half since 1990, and maternal health is on the global policy agenda like never before. Politicians have been getting the message, and governments across Africa and Asia have made big promises. Our role now is to hold them to account and make sure those promises become a reality. Join us, to make sure they deliver for women, at www.whiteribbonalliance.org.

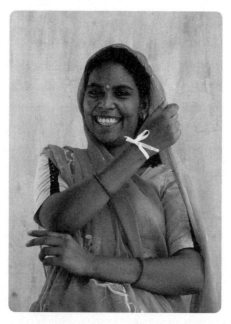

White Ribbon Alliance member, India

White Ribbon Alliance is a 501(c)(3) organization.
UK Charity Number 1143376 (registered 15 August 2011)

ABOUT THE

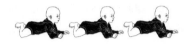

STAR SHOWERS CAMPAIGN

In November 2013, Daphne Oz, host of ABC's popular daytime TV programme *The Chew*, launched "Star Showers", an exciting new kind of baby shower – one in support of moms-to-be the world over. Daphne was joined by Hilaria Baldwin, Georgina Bloomberg, Georgina Chapman, Amber Sabathia and Latham Thomas in a special event to honour her approaching motherhood, but to honour much more too.

For millions of women around the world, giving birth is still one of the most dangerous things they might do, even though today at least ninety percent of childbirth deaths are preventable. Too many mothers-to-be kiss their families goodbye when they go into labour, knowing that there is a terrible chance they might never see their loved ones again.

That's where Star Showers comes in.

White Ribbon Alliance is asking friends and relatives to consider giving a donation to Star Showers via www.StarShowers.org at the same time as giving their friend a gift.

"Being part of Star Showers is like being part of a baby shower for the world where we are all celebrating and uniting for something bigger," said Daphne. "It's a powerful feeling of global sisterhood when we join together to make birth safe for women everywhere."

To find out how to be a part of showering *every* mother with love, visit www.whiteribbonalliance.org. You'll be able to make a gift in honour of a mother-to-be, who will receive a message from Star Showers letting her know how you've shared the love.

> We all have a part to play in supporting those around the world who strive for change, so that together we can realize our shared goal of no woman dying needlessly as she brings another life into the world.
>
> – *Sarah Brown, Global Patron of White Ribbon Alliance*

THANKS AND ACKNOWLEDGEMENTS

This book has been a truly collective enterprise. It was my agent, Rebecca Winfield, who – determined to find a way to support White Ribbon Alliance – sparked the original idea. Juliet Mabey at Oneworld Publications fanned that spark, and Robin Dennis – an editor of vision and precision, generosity and creativity – coaxed it into life. Thanks also to Henry Jeffreys, Jennifer Abel Kovitz, Alan Bridger, Lamorna Elmer, Missi Smith and the rest of the team at Oneworld, who are now helping it to fly.

My friends and colleagues Theresa Shaver and Betsy McCallon at White Ribbon Alliance gave me the space and encouragement to take this on. Catherine Hester, Andrea Miles and Katy Woods also supported me with their ideas, warmth and enthusiasm. Anna Chancellor, Diana Quick, Gaby Roslin and Helen Lederer were there for us as ever while we launched the idea on International Women's Day. Frances Ganges, Frances Day-Stirk, Cathrin Jerie and Rachael Lockey at the International Confederation of Midwives were immensely helpful in making connections and contributions. Rose Mlay, Samuel Senfuka, Shabnam Shahnaz,

Samjhana Phuyal, Jennifer Woodside, Kiev Martin, Suzanne Stalls, Nicky Leap, Maureen McTeer and Maryam Zar were all extremely generous with their time and experience. Arianna Huffington has been wonderfully supportive, as has Donna Karan. Lucy and Pob Smith, Eliza Langdon and Guy Guerrini, Nick Dewey and Emily Eavis, Mandy Briggs, Misty Buckley and Reg Matheson – heartfelt thanks! Meanwhile, my sisters Fran, Lucy and Emily McConville have been simply the best.

Anna Wadsworth arrived like a visiting angel to organize me and help get the book off the ground. Hazel Sainsbury rode in like the cavalry as we faced the deadline!

And, in between, many friends and supporters, doulas and midwives, mothers and fathers, White Ribbon Alliance members and Champions, contributed their thoughts, experience and wisdom. Their names follow. Thank you all!

Contributors

Yeshaya Adler

Lizzy Agams (Mrs Chinwe Akachi-Odoemene, BSc) of White Ribbon Alliance Nigeria

Priya Agrawal of Merck for Mothers (merckformothers.com)

Helen Atsma

Najmieh Batmanglij of Najmieh's Kitchen (najmiehskitchen.com)

Ionela Bodrug

Mandy Briggs

Kate Brown of Tell Me a Good Birth Story (tellmeagoodbirthstory.com)

Janet Chawla of MATRIKA (matrika-india.org)

Annie Clarke, nurse-midwife

Gorma "Mother Dear" Cole of the Bong County Reproductive Health Office, Liberia

Eleanor Copp, nurse-midwife (relaxedparenting.co.uk)

Sharlene Daly, midwife

Frances Day-Stirk, president of the International Confederation of Midwives (internationalmidwives.org)

Nancy Dennis

Emily Eavis of Glastonbury Festival (glastonburyfestivals.co.uk)

Michael Eavis of Glastonbury Festival (glastonburyfestivals.co.uk)

Robin Fink of Jungle Mamas, Pachamama Alliance (pachamama.org)

Carrie Lee Ferguson

Sarah Ferguson, Duchess of York

Jenn Forget of the International Confederation of Midwives (internationalmidwives.org)

Emma Freud

Rebecca Front

Dr Saraswathy Ganapathy of the Belaku Trust (belakutrust.org)

Sarah Goldsworthy

Dora Gouveia

Paige Grant

Hamish Guerrini

Gouri Guha of Peppery Thoughts (gouriguha.blogspot.com)

Kathy Herschderfer, midwife

Catherine Hester of White Ribbon Alliance

Stacia Smales Hill of Doula UK (doula.org.uk)

Milli Hill of the Positive Birth Movement (positivebirthmovement.org)

Katy Hope

Maggie Howell of Intuition Un Ltd (natalhypnotherapy.co.uk)

Arianna Huffington of *Huffington Post* (huffingtonpost.com/news/third-metric)

Sarah Javaid of MADE in Europe (madeineurope.org.uk)

Afande Jephrace (interviewed by the Belaku Trust)

Deepa Jha of White Ribbon Alliance India

Wakako Kai of the Japanese Organization for International Cooperation in Family Planning (joicfp.or.jp)

Lennie Kamwendo of White Ribbon Alliance Malawi

Donna Karan of Urban Zen Foundation (urbanzen.org)

Dr Radha Karnad

Zora King

Dina Sintadewi Landini of White Ribbon Alliance

Hannah Latham of *We Are Family* magazine (wearefamilymagazine. co.uk)

Larry Liza of Petals of Poetry (larryliza.blogspot.co.uk)

Rachael Lockey of the International Confederation of Midwives (international midwives.org)

Jody Lori of the University of Michigan School of Nursing

Chiku Lweno-Aboud of Mama Ye! (mamaye.org)

Julie Lys of the Canadian Nurses Association (canadian-nurse.com)

Kiev Martin of the American College of Nurse Midwives (midwife.org)

Reg Matheson

Davina McCall

Cass McNamara

Natalie Meddings of Tell Me a Good Birth Story (tellmeagoodbirth-story.com)

Rose Mlay of White Ribbon Alliance Tanzania

Fred Musoke of the Community Health Empowerment Organization, Luwero

Georgina Nortey of White Ribbon Alliance Ghana

Merry Ify Obah of White Ribbon Alliance Nigeria

Dr Srihartati Pandi of White Ribbon Alliance Indonesia

Rebecca Pasipanodya of White Ribbon Alliance Zimbabwe

Lesley Paulette of the Fort Smith Health and Social Services Authority, Northwest Territories, Canada

Samjhana Phuyal

Michelle Pino, nurse-midwife

Georgie Pope of Sound Travels (soundtravelsltd.com)

Lindy Roy of Yoga Māla (yogamala.co.uk)

Tosin Saraki of White Ribbon Alliance Nigeria and Wellbeing Foundation Africa (wbfafrica.org)

Bill Savage

Rebecca Schiller of Birthrights (birthrights.org.uk)

Samuel Senfuka, a chief of the Buganda people, of White Ribbon Alliance Uganda

Dr Shabnam Shahnaz of White Ribbon Alliance Bangladesh

Theresa Shaver of White Ribbon Alliance

Dr Rajendra Sharma

Esther Sikote (interviewed by the Belaku Trust)

André Simões

Katy Smith

Suzanne Stalls of the American College of Nurse Midwives (midwife. org)

Cathrine Streeval

Amy Szabo of Friends of Edna's Maternity Hospital (friendsofedna.org)

Dr Rebecca Tortello

Jelena Vulinovic-Zlatan

Vera Waters of the Interfaith Foundation (interfaithfoundation.org)

Sara Weinstein of Weinstein Carnegie Philanthropic Group (weinstein-pg.com)

Matthew Wood

Maryam Zar of Womenfound (womenfound.org) and the Fistula Foundation (fistulafoundation.org)

ART CREDITS

courtesy of the British Library International Dunhuang Project (p. 54)

Monk creating sand *mandala* © copyright Artur Bogacki/Shutterstock (p. 63)

A *vauva laatikko*, 1953, courtesy of the Työväenmuseo Werstas (Finnish Labour Museum Werstas) (p. 67)

Mother with baby, India, courtesy of White Ribbon Alliance (p. 80)

Midwife listening for the baby's heartbeat © copyright Liba Taylor and courtesy of the International Confederation of Midwives (p. 88)

Davina McCall with pregnant women in Malawi, courtesy of White Ribbon Alliance (p. 93)

Ancient Roman carving of midwife with mother, courtesy of Wellcome Images (p. 99)

Tapestry from Sarhua, Peru, courtesy of the Jean Isbell Andean Collection, Cornell University (p. 102)

Achuar women learning about pregnancy health, courtesy of Jungle Mamas, Pachamama (p. 109)

Carrie Lee and daughter Elle, courtesy of Carrie Lee Ferguson (p. 117)

Newborn blanketed in vernix © copyright Kati Molin/Shutterstock (p. 117)

Mother and baby moments after C-section delivery © copyright Steve Lovegrove/Shutterstock (p. 118)

Milli in the birthing pool with family, courtesy of Milli Hill (p. 118)

Baby's first words © copyright Liba Taylor and courtesy of the International Confederation of Midwives (p. 123)

Arabic "welcome" © copyright emran/Shutterstock (p. 124)

A Māori *ipu whenua*, or placenta bowl, courtesy of Wellcome Images (p. 126)

Inked foot prints in delivery room © copyright Liba Taylor and courtesy of the International Confederation of Midwives (p. 132)

Sleeping baby in grandmother's arms, France © copyright Paul Prescott/Shutterstock (p. 142)

Elder with baby, Burkina Faso © copyright Hector Conesa/Shutter-stock (p. 143)

Grandmother celebrating her grandchild, Nepal © copyright Paul Pres-cott/Shutterstock (p. 145)

Arrente baby smoking ceremony scenes © copyright Rachael Lockey and courtesy of the International Confederation of Midwives (p. 156)

New mother learning how to breastfeed, India © copyright Liba Taylor and courtesy of the International Confederation of Mid-wives (p. 163)

Getting the positioning right © copyright phloxii/Shutterstock (p. 162)

A *beschuit en muisjes* © copyright Ulrike de Haas (flickr.com/food-inthepicture) (p. 167)

A *cohen* blesses a baby before his naming ceremony © copyright Yehuda Boltshauser/Shutterstock (p. 173)

Mother and baby, India, courtesy of White Ribbon Alliance (p. 187)

New mothers showing off their babies, courtesy of White Ribbon Alliance (p. 190)

Babies and wrestlers face off in the *dohyō* and At the *Nakizumo* festival © Yoshikazu Tsuno/AFP/Getty Images (p. 195 and 196)

Sleep, baby © copyright Suzanne Taylor/Shutterstock (p. 198)

Mother carrying baby with *kanga*, Burkina Faso © copyright africa924/Shutterstock (p. 203)

Mother providing "kangaroo care", Rwanda, courtesy White Ribbon Alliance (p. 204)

Kanga ujumbe details © copyright David Inglesfield (p. 206 and 207)

Kanga draped over baby, Tanzania, courtesy of Chiku Lweno-Aboud (p. 207)

Baby's first bath © copyright negativkz/Shutterstock (p. 227)

Victorian christening gown © copyright lynea/Shutterstock (p. 232)

Shaving baby's hair as part of *aqiqah*, Malaysia,© copyright Ezz Mika Elya/Shutterstock (p. 234)

Samjhana and her daughter, courtesy of Samjhana Phuyal (p. 241)

Baby in basket cot, Nepal © copyright Paul Prescott/Shutterstock (p. 242)

Tedak siten ceremony scenes, Indonesia © copyright De Visu/Shutterstock (p. 251)

El Colacho jumping over infants © copyright Denis Doyle/Getty Images (p. 256)

At the Baba Umer *dargah* (shrine), India © copyright Tanzeel Rehman/Barcroft Media India/Getty Images (p. 258)

Baby posed for *doljabi* portrait © copyright Jamsong (p. 261)

Mother and baby, Burkina Faso, courtesy White Ribbon Alliance (p. 266)

Infant held by many hands © copyright Chris Curtis/Shutterstock (p. 268)

White Ribbon Alliance member, India, courtesy White Ribbon Alliance (p. 270)

INDEX

ABOUT THE AUTHOR

Brigid McConville is a director of White Ribbon Alliance. An award-winning journalist and filmmaker, she is the author most recently of *Stories of Mothers Lost*. When she is not travelling the world to ensure WRA's mission that pregnancy and childbirth are safe for all, she splits her time between London and Somerset.